Yoga for Equestrians

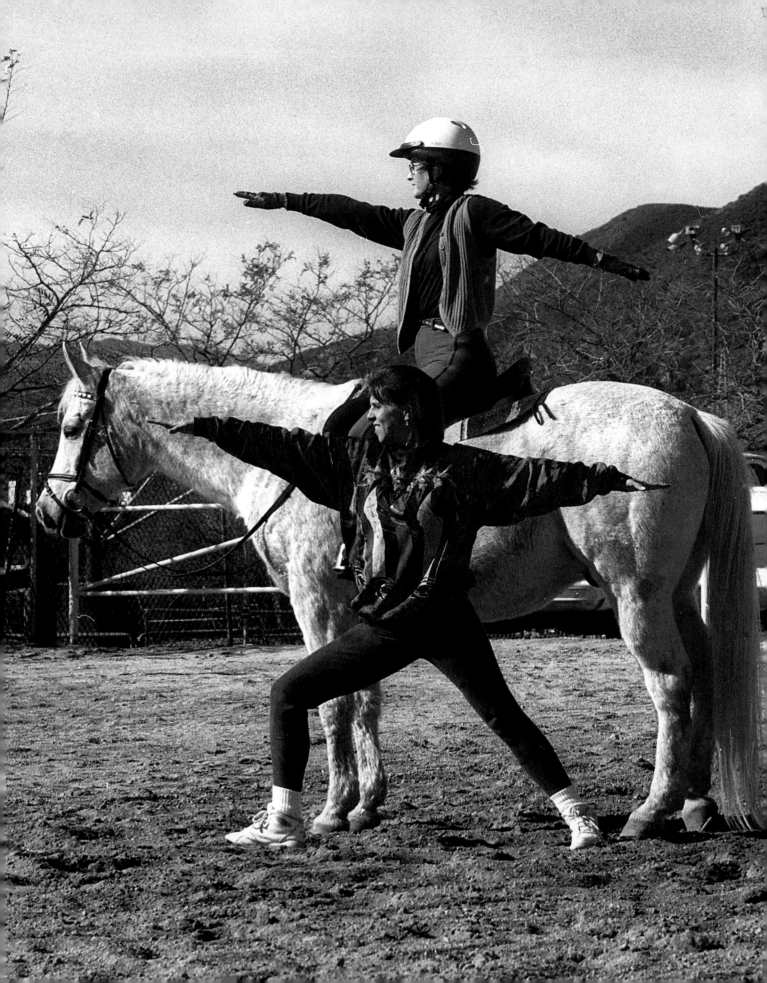

YOGA FOR EQUESTRIANS

A New Path for
Achieving Union with the Horse

Linda Benedik and Veronica Wirth

TRAFALGAR SQUARE PUBLISHING

NORTH POMFRET, VERMONT

First published in 2000 by
Trafalgar Square Publishing
North Pomfret, Vermont 05053

Reprinted 2001, 2002, 2003, 2004 and 2007

Printed in China by 1010 International Printing LTD

Disclaimer of Liability:
The authors and publisher shall have neither liability nor responsibility to any person or entity with respect to any loss or damage caused or alleged to be caused directly or indirectly by the information contained in this book. While the book is as accurate as the authors can make it, there may be errors, omissions, and inaccuracies.

Library of Congress Cataloging-in-Publication Data
Benedik, Linda.
    Yoga for equestrians : a new path for achieving union with the horse / Linda Benedik and Veronica Wirth.
        p.cm.
        Includes bibliographical references (p.).
        ISBN 1-57076-136-1 (pbk.)
    1. Horsemanship—Psychological aspects. 2. Yoga. I. Wirth, Veronica. II. Title.

SF309.B464 2000
798.2'01'9—dc21   9-087512
ISBN 978-1-57076-136-2

10 9 8 7 6
Line illustrations by Veronica Wirth
Photography by Linda Benedik

Contents

✧

About the Authors

By Linda Benedik, BA

An important lesson that horses teach equestrians of any style, any level is that there is always more to learn about riding. A rider for over thirty years, my passion for the art and discipline of dressage has flourished since I was a young girl growing up in the beautiful Maryland horse country. A graduate of the Lake Erie College Equestrian Studies program of Ohio, my work has led me to teach on both East and West coasts and establish the Harmony With Horses Balanced Riding Program of Southern California in 1994. For nearly two decades I've experienced tremendous satisfaction as a trainer and instructor, yet I continue to learn as a student of the horse with each passing day.

Aside from typical horse-related activities such as shoveling, grooming, and "weight lifting" (feed bags, rubber mats, water buckets, etc.), and before including yoga practice in my routine, for many years riding was the *only* physical exercise I was committed to. Since much of my life has been spent in the saddle, maintaining virtually the same body position for countless hours on innumerable horses, I came to recognize certain physical habits that resulted from riding—some that contributed to my health, others that did not.

Years of riding had contributed to stiffness and a restricted range of movement in distinct areas of my body. When evaluated for fitness at a local YMCA, my flexibility tested poorly and this nearly convinced me that I was in terrible shape...until I performed the "Harvard Step Test." This three-minute step exercise measured cardio-respiratory endurance and my resulting heart rate indicated I was in fine physical condition and cardiac health. The examiners wanted to know what I did to stay in shape.

"I ride horses," I replied.

"No...what do you do for *exercise*?" they asked.

When I reiterated that my entire physical program was dedicated to riding horses, these fitness "experts" were in disbelief. I've encountered this common misconception throughout my life—some people believe that riding horses is not aerobic. The results of my fitness evaluation certainly proved that the opposite was true. While stepping to the beat of a metronome, I had consciously regulated my breathing rhythm correspondingly. This aerobic activity was similar to the rhythmical breathing I used while schooling horses actively at trot or canter—for periods much longer than three minutes! Using proper breathing techniques while riding had increased my aerobic endurance and improved my physical condition. This reaffirmed my conviction that breathing in rhythm with movement is key to successful riding.

Breathing is recognized by equestrian professionals as fundamental to riding and many trainers direct their students to "*Breathe, breathe!*" but very few are able to teach them *how*. Like most students, I was *never* taught breathing techniques in a riding lesson—I learned them in another "arena." During my training as a singer and musician, I was instructed in correct abdominal breathing and learned the important link between rhythm, breath, movement, and relaxation. Establishing a relaxed rhythm while playing music enabled me to do so in the saddle and powerful, breath-supported singing really strengthened my abdominal muscles. These skills have helped me to produce steady, rhythmical gaits in the horses I ride and have been integrated into my teaching.

My experience as a riding teacher has strengthened my belief that correct breathing should be the *first* lesson introduced to the rider. Over the years, I have noticed an overwhelming lack of knowledge regarding correct breathing techniques in equestrians of all levels. When asked to take a deep breath, many riders draw their shoulders up toward their ears and hollow out their abdomens—visible signs of incorrect breathing. It became obvious to me that riders would greatly benefit from learning how to consciously master rhythmical, abdominal breathing *before* getting on a horse. Because sitting on a horse can be distracting or generate fear, anxiety, or nervousness, breathing is best addressed first on the ground to foster relaxation, focus, and technique. To encourage this, I introduced Yoga for Equestrians to my riding students as the perfect complement to mounted work. I had practiced yoga and knew its conscious, deep breathing and gentle stretching exercises would enhance a rider's flexibility both in and out of the saddle.

Yoga soon became a popular and integral part of the Harmony With Horses program—preparing students in body and mind for riding. In 1996, I asked Veronica, a fellow dressage enthusiast, rider, and yoga practitioner, to present a Yoga for Equestrians workshop as part of a clinic that included both unmounted and mounted classes. The combination of Veronica's knowledge of Hatha and Kundalini yoga, and her riding experience was perfect for introducing the benefits of yoga to a varied group of Western, English, and dressage riders. After a morning of unmounted work, the participants all showed significant improvements in their riding that afternoon. With increased relaxation, flexibility, and focus, these riders achieved direct, observable results on their horses. Even for those auditing, the benefits of integrating yoga with riding were clear.

This presentation of Yoga for Equestrians was the first of many, and I remain eternally grateful to Veronica for her valuable contributions to the Harmony With Horses Balanced Riding Program and for the wonderful insights into yoga that grace the pages of this book. She has taught me ways to improve my own flexibility, and her compassionate, sensitive nature has tempered my life with a powerful feminine energy, enabling me to become *flexible* in more ways than one. In a gentle, intuitive manner, Veronica shares her gifts in a soothing, melodic tone very conducive to deep relaxation and stillness.

My sincerest thanks and appreciation to you, Veronica, for your close friendship and for helping me to grow and expand as an individual, teacher, and rider. We've laughed, learned, cried, dreamed, brainstormed, even sung together! Our collaboration and the multitude of experiences we've shared have greatly contributed to the tapestry of my life and to my deeper understanding and practice of yoga.

For all students of the horse, this book can be a valuable guide and may even transform your approach to riding. I am pleased to share my insights into riding and offer a fresh perspective toward understanding and applying the classical principles of horsemanship. This book is not just another how-to guide, nor does it merely trot out a trendy new fad. Rather, it introduces a comprehensive, holistic program for rider development involving the practical integration of yoga to help you achieve your goals. My riding students have progressed more rapidly than ever before and you, too, can integrate Yoga for Equestrians into your riding repertoire to reap its many rewards.

The riding theory and language should be familiar, but the description of new riding *tools*—alternative ideas and techniques to help you achieve traditional goals—may be unfamiliar. Holistic riding involves more than physical mechanics and cultivates a deeper connection between body, breath, mind, and horse. As you explore this program, I suggest you bring an open mind and a committed desire to improve: to be the best rider you can be. The horses you ride deserve your increased attention to Self, so that your communication with them is clearer, more receptive, and more compassionate.

Remember, on your journey strive to remain clear and present in each moment, keep your eyes, heart, and mind open to your riding future and the possibilities it holds...achieving Union with the horse is a tangible reality that can truly be yours.

Happy Riding! *Namaste*

By Veronica Wirth

As a rider, I have come to appreciate what yoga has to offer in many ways. When I began practicing Hatha yoga after being injured in a car accident, I was amazed and delighted to find that doing just a few simple postures each day virtually eliminated the pain and discomfort in my back and neck that I had been struggling with for months afterward. At that time, I had been riding horses for about two years and was just beginning to fall in love with dressage. My injuries were most troublesome when I was in the saddle and my body developed very creative "evasions" to protect my back, inhibiting my movement as I struggled to effectively ride the big, rolling movements of my horse. Yoga made it comfortable to ride again, suppling and strengthening my body as it helped restore my balance and symmetry.

But yoga has touched me in other ways as well. Pursuing riding as an adult who had been on one too many terrifying trail rides as a youngster, I found myself facing fears I thought I had long got over. During this time in my life, I was also exploring the spiritual side of myself and, in 1993, I took up meditation and Kundalini yoga, a type of yoga that focuses strongly on breathing techniques and energy movement. Some years later, there was an instance while riding when I felt my old fears rising up again. The horse immediately picked up on my tenseness, and I could feel our connection starting to spiral out of control. Without consciously thinking about it, I began to breathe deeply and draw my awareness to the center of my body, just as I had done many times in yoga practice. I had the sensation of all the scattered pieces of myself being drawn to my center like a magnet by way of my breath. Within a couple of strides, the horse began quieting underneath me. I was amazed! Not only had I been able to regain my focus in that moment, but I had prevented my fear from taking control of my actions. It happened not by fighting my fear, but by moving *through* it in a new and more effective way. Practicing yoga over time has positively affected my riding by increasing my awareness, teaching me how to more easily establish and hold my focus and enabling me to deal with my fears much more effectively.

When Linda approached me to teach yoga to her riding students at her workshop in 1996, I had no idea that we would, a short time after, begin collaboration on a book together. That workshop was truly a catalyst for me and my riding. Although I was familiar with the effectiveness of yoga through my own experience, nothing prepared me for the overwhelmingly positive effect it had on the students' rides that day. It was Linda's vision that crystallized how yoga could directly and profoundly influence the art of riding. Our lives have not been the same since!

I offer my deepest gratitude to Linda, my partner on this extraordinary journey. An extremely gifted rider and trainer who has long been ahead of her time, she brings refreshing levels of creativity, integrity, and passion to her teaching not often seen in the horse world. Not only has she transformed my own riding, but I never cease to be moved as I watch her transform her students' riding in the same way. Her knowledge, enthusiasm, and dedication to the art of riding form the heart of this book.

Linda, thank you from my heart for being a great and true friend. Your dynamic nature inspires me to always reach further and push my edges. Your confidence and deep sense of commitment inspire me to never say never! Thank you for your courage, determination, and unending support of my work and my expression, and, most of all, for being who you are.

Today, after riding since 1987 and practicing yoga since 1990, I enjoy sharing what has worked for me and what I continue to discover in my own work with horses, with equestrians and non-equestrians alike. Certified as a Hatha yoga teacher, I now guide others in ways to use their breath to become more aware of their bodies, thoughts, and emotions, encouraging them to nurture their intuition and listen to their body as they become more in tune with their own natural wisdom.

The process of bringing this book into being has, in its own way, been a form of yoga. It has been a process of discovery. I've encountered various polarities within myself: activity and stillness, holding on and releasing, pushing through and yielding. As we worked on this book, I learned to remind myself of the very things that I say so often to my students: "Come back to center," "Be in the present moment," and *"Breathe!"*

I have, within the limitations of print, done my best to imbue the yoga in these pages with the sense of joy, wonder, and discovery that I have found on my own path through yoga, as I continue to discover the deep, inherent intelligence of the body. I have found that our bodies hold an incredible wealth of wisdom for us to discover, and yoga is one of the best ways to help unlock it. The greatest gift I can give is to share with you the templates which have helped me uncover this wisdom, and the enjoyment, satisfaction, and sense of wonder born out of that process. As you travel through this book, I encourage you to strive to make yoga *your own* by approaching it with the pure delight and creativity of a child. The photos and directives on these pages are guidelines to start you on your journey. Where you go is up to you! May your journey enhance your enthusiasm and love for riding and bring you closer to Union, not only with the horses you ride, but to your most valuable teacher and dearest friend—your Self.

From my heart—the spirit in me honors the spirit in you! *Namaste*

PART I

The Journey Begins

"True riding mastery can only be reached by the person who, for years and years, has kept his mind open to new ideas, and even he should always be prepared to admit that there is still much to be learned." [1]
WILHELM MÜSELER, *Riding Logic*

CHAPTER ONE

About this Book

The Program

Our unique approach merges two very ancient disciplines—horsemanship and yoga—and presents Yoga for Equestrians as a practical, beneficial, and enjoyable program to enhance your riding skills. Yoga integrated with horsemanship teaches and produces desirable rider qualities such as enhanced awareness, flexibility, balance, and correct breathing in rhythm with movement, all of which generate a relaxed focus in the rider's performance.

The concepts and techniques presented in this book are tried and true and consistently reflected in our students' easy, steady progress in both unmounted and mounted work. Yoga practice complements any mounted training program and greatly enhances each rider's journey toward Union with the horse.

The Book

Yoga for Equestrians is written for the equestrian, riding student, and riding teacher in every style or discipline. Whether you ride Western or English or jump, event, or do dressage; whether you ride for recreation, pleasure, competition, self-discovery, or artistic expression—if you wish to honor your horse and are open to new possibilities on how to accomplish that, this book is for you. It has been specifically designed to benefit the rider, fulfill a rider's needs, and assist in achieving rider goals. In Part I, The Journey Begins, you will be introduced to our program and discover the similarities between the ancient traditions of yoga and horsemanship. You will learn what yoga is, and what it is not. Our students enthusiastically share some of their accomplishments and reflect on Yoga for Equestrians. We discuss the many ways yoga can benefit you as an equestrian and offer explicit guidelines for practice.

In Part II, The Foundations of Union, we examine some of the key concepts and important principles upon which our program is founded. To truly appreciate Yoga for Equestrians, it is important to understand the framework upon which this sturdy structure relies. You will find that our approach is rooted in ancient wisdom. For equestrians

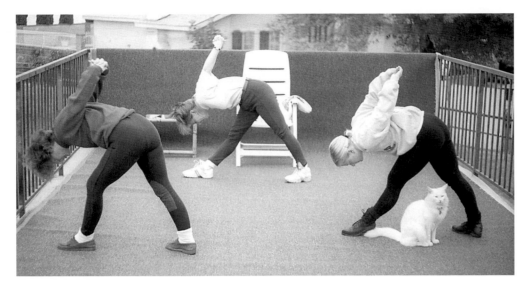

Teaching gentle stretches and correct breathing techniques, Yoga for Equestrians is a practical and enjoyable way to address your individual riding goals.

hungry for knowledge, eager for new ways to get results, yet patient enough to build their own, long-lasting foundation as a rider, we bring this wisdom into the light.

Part II examines how the power of your mind can help you accomplish your goals and create positive changes in your life. By tapping into the potential of your subconscious mind, you can make significant improvements to your riding and enhance your yoga practice. To understand how your subconscious mind can help you, we introduce *meditation*✳ and *visualization*✳ as effective rider tools. We also explore the significance of what it means to become a *"conscious rider"*✳ and look at the benefits of riding without force. We define *rhythmic stillness*✳, an *altered state*✳ of mind achieved when an accomplished rider, through *rhythm*✳, breathing, and movement, merges with the horse; in rhythmic stillness, horse and rider become One.

We also present the first series of yoga positions or *asanas*✳, a group of rhythmic poses that help you learn how to breathe in rhythm with movement, and introduce you to *pranayama*✳, yogic breathing exercises that teach awareness and control of your breath. Breathing skills are essential for equestrians to move in rhythmic harmony with the horse, yet most riders need to become conscious of this inherent ability.

Part III, Yoga for Equestrians, consists of three chapters which correspond to distinct divisions of your body: the mid-section or *center*✳, the lower body, and the upper body. Each chapter discusses the ideal functioning of these areas in achieving a *balanced seat*✳ and provides pertinent anatomical insights and detailed information to assist you in understanding the role of your body in relation to the horse.

Part IV, The Journey Continues, presents yoga routines in durations of five, ten, or twenty minutes of practice. Yoga is a transportable and practical activity to assist you in warming up before riding, so we offer routines you can do at home, work, at the stable, and even at a show or competition. Part IV also presents yoga cool-downs that can be performed at the stable after an arduous ride. You can comfortably perform these routines in riding attire, as our students do, and eventually, you can customize your own routines based on individual needs and preferences. The final chapter presents a special program of Yoga in the Saddle, intended to be performed with the help of an assistant or trainer.

The models used to illustrate the asanas are students who practice yoga and ride regularly. Because most of us, whether novice or advanced, experience varying degrees of flexibility, the photographs depict a range of possibilities that illustrate that riders should consider themselves a "work-in-progress": always moving forward toward their goals. Our models may not always achieve the deepest, ultimate yoga postures, but the photographs confirm that each individual's practice of yoga is appropriate to his or her abilities. Use the photographs as reference points as you find your own place within each pose.

We recommended that you read through Parts I and II before commencing your practice of Yoga for Equestrians. The preliminary chapters provide background and ideas to reflect upon and helpful information you will need to be familiar with before you begin. At the end of each section, you will find relevant asanas, grouped together for your convenience. Throughout the book, terms designated by a "✱" symbol are defined in the Glossary, Appendix 1, located in the back of the book for easy reference.

Our dearest hope is that you truly enjoy your yoga practice and that it enhances your equestrian journey. May Yoga for Equestrians expand your awareness and your riding repertoire and fill you with a greater compassion for yourself and the horses you ride.

Why Yoga?

Horses around the world speak a common language that is clear, uncomplicated, direct, and, for the most part, silent. They rely primarily on a language of body movements, expressions, and postures. Using the body to communicate is one of the first lessons the horse teaches *any* person learning to ride. *This is the essence of riding and a rider's most challenging task.*

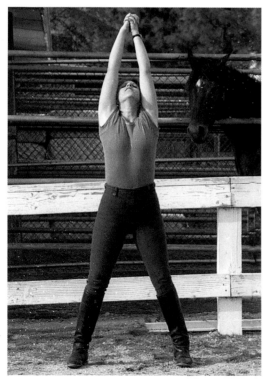

*Yoga **feels good** and is a treat for your body and mind.*

Why yoga? We live in a time of necessary healing of the relationships we share with each other, the earth, and all living things. Leaders in the equestrian community have begun to really listen to the horse and, as a result, are adapting their riding and training techniques to reflect a gentler, more humane, and compassionate attitude. This "higher" thinking is becoming more widespread, and the success stories speak for themselves, even to non-equestrians! It is not difficult to recognize an animal that trusts its handler and enjoys working with its rider in an environment of respect and cooperation, as opposed to a horse that has been beaten into submission and obeys out of fear. Creating a deep bond of trust, communication, and synchronicity between horse and rider may sound like an almost magical achievement, yet you can create such a connection with the horse and grow to understand the true meaning of *Union*✱.

Yoga for Equestrians contributes to this evolution of higher thought and practice. It will prompt you to spend time working independently, taking the initiative and assuming greater responsibility for your improvement and growth as a rider. Yoga practice is a way for you to honor the horse by striving to become the best rider you can be. The horse, in turn, will reflect the positive changes in you by becoming more willing, balanced, and pleasurable to ride.

Bear in mind that the concepts we present here are not "new"; in fact, they are as ancient and classical as horsemanship itself. Yet to many riders these ideas may *feel* new or different. That's okay! Regardless of any ambitions or competitive goals you have for your equestrian sport or steadfast principles your trainer enforces during lessons, remember that your equestrian journey is your own. We invite you to branch out from the more traditional methods you may be accustomed to and explore these principles. Yoga practice will complement and enhance the comparatively brief time you spend working on your riding skills in the saddle. Why yoga? Because it works...and we will show you how. We encourage you to make Yoga for Equestrians a part of your life.

Parallels: Yoga and Riding

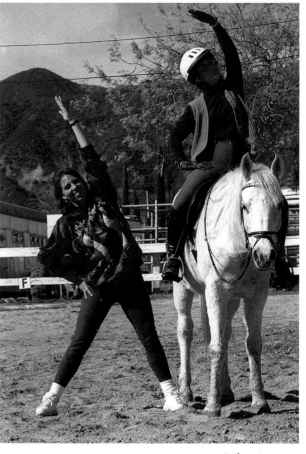

Riding **is** *yoga!*

- Classical horsemanship and traditional yoga are very ancient practices. Both originated thousands of years ago and, in their purest form, encourage learning through compassion, kindness, and awareness. The earliest known surviving work on the art of riding was a very detailed treatise written over twenty-three centuries ago by Xenophon, a Greek soldier and master horseman. His humane methods reflect a foundation built on intuition, kindness, and compassion toward the horse. [2] The practice of yoga will inspire you to treat your body and the horse in the same manner. Rather than forcing or implementing ruthless training methods, yoga teaches you to allow, listen closely, and gently coax.

- Within both practices, it is common to find that the more you learn, the more you realize how much there is to know...the scope of knowledge is endless! Learning to ride is an ongoing process; the principles and practices of horsemanship are continuously evolving. With roots that date back thousands of years, both yoga and riding are timeless studies that involve journeys of self-discovery and growth.

- Both yoga and riding integrate breathing with moving in rhythm. Riding is a rhythmic activity in which the rider flows synchronously and in concert with the movements of the horse. To "dance" with an equine partner, the rider must breathe and move in a relaxed and consistent rhythm. Through rhythmic poses and controlling the rhythm of breath, yoga brings heightened awareness to the movements of your body. Breath control connects and guides your movements in both riding and yoga.

- Riding and yoga are activities that engage both mind and body, stimulating you to identify and explore your limitations—physically and mentally. Yoga provides an ideal forum in which you can learn to safely and gradually stretch your limitations without injury or discomfort by heightening your awareness and ability to focus. While riding also involves the gradual development of these skills, your ability to work beyond your limits can be honed through yoga practice, then transferred to your riding with greater ease.

- Correct training methods provide a foundation for the horse by cultivating balance, suppleness, flexion, and mental focus over time. In the same manner, yoga develops these fundamental qualities in the rider, who can then become more effective in the saddle. A strong foundation of balance, flexibility, and focus enables both horse and rider to progress more competently into their desired riding discipline.

- Yoga practice enhances awareness of your body's symmetry, while also revealing your imbalances. The horse provides much the same feedback for the rider who has learned to listen and understand the horse through the *mirroring*∗ phenomenon (discussed in Chapter 5).

- Yoga and riding share the universal goal of establishing union. In yoga, "union" refers to merging all aspects of yourself, attaining unity of body, mind, and spirit. When we learn to foster wholeness within ourselves through yoga, we explore the very techniques that enable us to achieve Union with the horse. There are many similarities between riding and yoga...it is quite natural to consider that riding *is* yoga!

Our Students Share

Apryl Knobbe

Apryl Knobbe, a 29-year-old digital artist who works on major motion pictures, sits for long hours in front of a computer, dealing with deadlines and stressful working conditions. Apryl became aware that many of her riding challenges resulted from how she spent her time at work; in her own words, *"slouching and non-moving."* Apryl reports, *"It's hard to keep my posture on the horse and I don't have much strength in my legs...it really bothered me, at first, to ride because I'd get cramps and be sore for a few days."*

Apryl describes the benefits of yoga practice: *"Yoga prepares me to get on the horse. It calms me down and I can forget everything else, just get up and enjoy myself relaxing and being receptive. I used to try too hard to both calm down and control the horse. I would think constantly, 'Okay, what am I doing wrong?' instead of just listening to myself and feeling what's right. Now, I listen to the horse and listen to myself to see what feels natural."*

Yoga has assisted Apryl in positively modifying her riding habits. She states, *"I really don't get sore at all anymore and my joints don't ache as much as they used to after I ride. My balance is a lot better and I can keep my feet in the stirrups much easier now! Not only have the stretches prevented my hips, legs, and joints from hurting, but what is really amazing to me is the fact that I no longer lose my balance. This is a big improvement for me; my balance was all over the place at first and difficult to maintain. I believe it's the yoga that has really been helping me to learn to keep my balance and feel what the horse is doing."*

Anna Ruth Souza

Anna Ruth is a 40-year-old law office administrator who has been riding a little over a year. She shares, *"I am very much right-handed. I knew I wasn't ambidextrous, but I realize now [as a rider] that I do need to use the left side of my body. I'm trying as I eat—I switch my fork so that I can get more use out of my left hand. I also do things at work with my left side a little bit more than I used to."*

Yoga was instrumental in helping Anna Ruth become more symmetrical although she was initially skeptical and not very interested in the practice of yoga. She explains, *"I'd never been a big yoga person. My perception of yoga was that it was sort of 'way out there.' As far as I'm concerned, the yoga that we do related to the equestrian is not that. It's very helpful because I have a direction for it: to help me ride the horse better. Yoga is something I've never been interested in before, but I just tried it. I was very surprised the first time that I enjoyed it. I think that's why I still am interested in it. I find that I like it when I do it. I like the stretches most of all. I've been doing them a lot at home, in the morning. I am incorporating yoga into my everyday life."*

When asked how yoga has changed her riding, Anna Ruth responded: *"It's improved my balance, it's completely improved my breathing, my endurance, and relaxation on the horse. I think it's helped overall, in every aspect. This program is purposeful, it's directed toward riding. I think it's very helpful and I enjoy it tremendously."*

Virginia Hildreth

Like many riders, Virginia, a 51-year-old creative director for a real estate newspaper, spends her day sitting for long periods of time. *"I forget that I have a body when I sit in front of a computer the entire day. Because I do nothing but brain work, honoring and allowing my body is an issue I'm working on. Riding has helped me to think of myself as whole...and yoga awakens my body to being alive."*

Virginia explains, *"I wanted to learn how to trust my own physical sensations, letting my body awareness be my guide, as opposed to leading with my mind into the world. Integrating yoga with riding has opened up my eyes to a whole different approach to life—I knew I had to integrate all of the elements of my Self to become balanced. I had been relating to the world with too much 'brain,' living too much up in my head. I had to find a way to change. Since I've always loved horses, it seemed like a natural entry into a world that is unspoken, learning a physical activity which required less analytical thought, more emotion and feeling."*

Virginia's practice even includes grooming the horse and tacking. She shares, *"I use yoga when I'm tacking up. I relax into what I'm doing, which I've learned from yoga. When I curry, there are places on the horse's body where I lighten up and come back, it's this flow and ebb that we do with each other before I ride that is part of yoga. You stretch, you hold, you release, and you breathe the whole time."*

As an adult beginner, Virginia relates, *"There are people, especially women, who are riding just because they love it. All their lives they've had the classical dream horse as part of their own personal myth, and now they're at the point where they have a choice to do something about it. To go through the traditional schooling—some of it is very superficial, very masculine, and it may not take you where you want to go. Sometimes it looks like you don't have a choice, which is why I had to find something else, because I wanted a choice. This program is about growth and it is a really safe, nurturing environment to do it in. At this point, I can't imagine not doing it."*

Amanda Deaton

Amanda, a 23-year-old tack shop owner, has been a competitive rider since age eight. *"I started out doing three-day eventing, then did jumpers, hunters, flat hunters, reining horses, Quarter-horse hunters, and Western pleasure horses."* Her show ring performance revealed,

"I've done really well in pleasure classes, hunter under saddle classes, you know, where they judge the horse. I've never done well in equitation classes."

To improve, Amanda felt she needed to eliminate *"old, and well-ingrained bad [riding] habits. I've got to keep those heels down, shoulders back, arch my back, elbows in, heels down, heels down...Way down! Are you in pain? Okay, you're doing it right!"*

We wondered if she had really been taught that if it hurt, it meant you were doing it right. Amanda replied, *"Not to that extent, but with the trainer that I rode with for the longest period of time, it was, 'Sit up straight. Keep your heels down. Heels down, heels down."* As a result of the familiar 'heels down' mantra, Amanda's ankles had become hyperflexed and weak. She remembers, *"...that 'heels down' thing was ingrained well into my brain."*

Amanda, too, had misconceptions about yoga. Never having tried it before, she believed *"that you moved around more and it was more like aerobics. I thought it involved quicker motions than the slow stretching and visualizing. I knew visualization was involved, but it was much more effective than I had pictured. I had read about visualizing, but when I tried it on the horse, I couldn't visualize anything. I couldn't put what I had read into use on a horse until I had done it during yoga; and I realized that visualization does work."*

Additionally, yoga assisted Amanda with rhythmical breathing while riding— something she did not learn from her trainers. She states, *"I knew to breathe from my center and not from my chest but that came from singing class. This rhythmical breathing, I learned through yoga. It has really made a big difference for me."*

Sarah Rose

Sarah is a 20-year-old student and a rider of fourteen years. She shares, *"Incorporating yoga into riding was a big turn-on for me because it was really different, I had never done it before and, by doing it, I became more aware of my body when riding. Instead of trying to lock myself into a set position that I thought was right, I just let myself go with the horse and balance naturally."*

Due to past injuries, Sarah faced physical challenges in her riding. She explains, *"Whenever a person gets an injury, they baby it and avoid working with it and just keep the area stiff. I've got problems with my shoulders, lower back, and my hips. Just having somebody tell me why I need to relax and loosen up, to be more mobile in those areas, has really helped. With yoga, the more you work with a certain part of your body, the more you are aware of it, the more you can control it, and it doesn't hurt anymore."*

There was another challenge Sarah faced that caused her to feel self-conscious. She shares, *"Getting my breathing going is difficult. Unmounted, it's okay, but mounted it's difficult because I tense up. Once I relax, especially when I do yoga before riding, it's a lot easier."* Sarah shares, *"The first time I was kind of embarrassed to actually do the breathing and stretch because I was self-conscious. But this friendly environment helped me to get over that almost instantly. Nobody is critical of you, everybody just wants you to do well."*

✦

CHAPTER TWO

Yoga Basics

SECTION 1. What is Yoga?

There is no concise textbook definition of yoga that satisfies everyone; this ancient tradition has been interpreted in a variety of ways by people throughout the world and throughout history. You may have already formulated your own personal interpretation of yoga or what it represents to you. To many, yoga is a *"way of life, an integrated system of education for the body, mind and inner spirit."* [4] To others, it is the perfect *"all purpose exercise."* [5] However, each definition of yoga refers to three essential elements:

- body, through which we experience the world physically;

- mind, responsible for our intellectual perceptions; and

- *soul*✶ or *spirit*✶, the unseen part of us that seeks balance and inner-peace in our lives.

The practice of yoga aids in the preservation of our health and well-being and creates inner harmony, enhancing our relationship to the world around us. Despite references to the soul, yoga is not a religion, but rather a practical approach to self-discovery.

The word yoga is an ancient *Sanskrit*✶ word that means "union" or to "make whole" and refers to the ultimate alliance between body, mind, and spirit. There are many systems of yoga. Like the spokes of a wheel that converge at the center, they provide numerous paths to the central goal of wholeness and balance.

The path most familiar to the Western world and the one this program is primarily based on is *Hatha yoga*✶. It is the avenue of yoga which seeks balance through toning and strengthening the physical body. Hatha (pronounced HA-ta), also a Sanskrit word, illuminates the many *polarities*✶ within each of us. These polarities are represented by the Sun (ha), which symbolizes *masculine energy*✶ expressed in the form of *activity*, and the Moon (tha),

"The unification of two things, whatever their nature, is called yoga." [3] A.G. MOHAN, Yoga for Body, Breath, and Mind

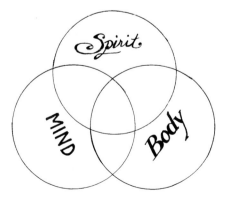

Yoga fosters union between mind, body, and spirit.

"There is nothing in yoga that competes with any religious orthodoxy or with any other system of belief. Rather, yoga is a vehicle for growth and development that anyone can adapt to one's own way of making life's journey." [6] A.G. MOHAN, *Yoga For Body, Breath, and Mind*

which symbolizes *feminine energy*✷ expressed in the form of *receptivity*. Both masculine and feminine energies are present in all men and women to varying degrees. Hatha yoga is a means to bring a balanced unity to the polarities within ourselves through asanas and pranayama, which are the foundation of Yoga for Equestrians.

Awareness

Yoga is a powerful method that cultivates self-awareness. To become self-aware is to truly know your mind and body and understand the relationship between the two. Your success as a rider relies greatly on your level of *body-mind*✷ awareness, which can improve through your practice of yoga.

Traditionally, a key function of the riding instructor has been to assist the student in developing body awareness in order to achieve the correct position on the horse. However, when equestrians take the initiative to improve body awareness off the horse, their performance on horseback is greatly enhanced. Even for advanced riders, the practice of yoga can expand self-awareness and promote a deeper connection with the horse.

A Stillness

"...yoga is not about adopting any particular set of beliefs, but about coming to know through your own experience. It is not about becoming the blind follower of anything, but about assisting you on your own chosen path." [7] A.G. MOHAN, *Yoga For Body, Breath, and Mind*

Yoga is a gentle way for the equestrian to move into *stillness*✷. To move into stillness is to quiet the internal chatter of your mind, accept your riding abilities, your learning process, and your body without harsh self-criticism or judgment. You will find this stillness more accessible when you have learned to be fully involved in the moment and fully attentive to your activity. When you establish stillness on the horse, you develop a *kinesthetic*✷ awareness, riding with more feel, breathing deeply in rhythm with your own movements and the horse's gaits. Stillness allows you to heed your instincts and the subtle feedback of your body, enabling you to develop a riding repertoire of stored kinesthetic sensations, or *body memories*✷. In stillness you can truly listen to and understand the horse.

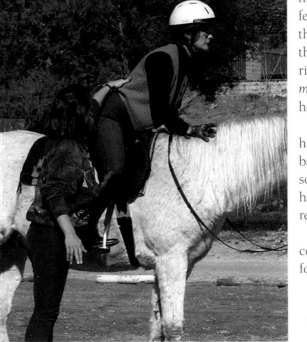

A riding instructor may be the only person who has ever assisted with your awareness of balance and alignment.

As riders, we must remain *centered*✷ and in harmony with the horse through every movement and every activity. Maintaining balance, stillness, and the ability to be fully present are important so that we are consistently able to perceive clearly what is happening. This allows us to choose the most appropriate responses to communicate effectively with the horse.

If the idea of achieving stillness seems paradoxical when considering the active physical nature of riding, consider the following metaphor by author Erich Schiffman:

"Imagine a spinning top. Stillness is like a perfectly centered top, spinning so fast it appears motionless. It appears this way not because it isn't moving, but because it's spinning at full speed. Stillness is not the absence or negation of energy, life, or movement. Stillness is dynamic. It is unconflicted movement, life in harmony

with itself, skill in action. It can be experienced whenever there is total, uninhibited, uncon-flicted participation in the moment you are in—when you are wholeheartedly present with whatever you are doing."[8]

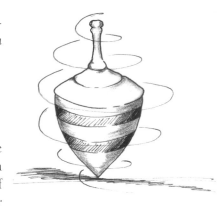

A Journey

Whatever your desired goal, the journey toward fulfilling it involves progressive movement. This movement occurs at your own pace and can be interspersed with periods of pause, or immobility. The ebb and flow between activity and rest in itself becomes an integral part of your journey. As you connect with your momentum, your activity becomes yoga. As you unite with your respite, your pause becomes yoga. When you fulfill a goal, when you experience a plateau in your riding, when you hold an asana and then release with mindful attention, each becomes part of your yoga practice and your journey. Self-understanding is possibly the most intricate journey of all. Let yoga serve as a guide on your inner journey as well as your equestrian journey toward Union.

Stillness is dynamic, like a perfectly centered top that spins so fast it appears motionless.

SECTION 2. The Benefits: Balance, Wholeness...Union

One of the unique benefits of Yoga for Equestrians is that it addresses the rider as a whole. It is a means for the rider to first attain unity of body, mind, and spirit, then ultimately integrate with the body, mind, and spirit of the horse to achieve Union. In contrast to other rider fitness regimens that primarily isolate the physical aspect of rider development (such as aerobics, weight training, or conditioning programs to improve muscular efficiency), yoga practice is *holistic*✳ as it addresses and balances the facets of your entire being—your *Self*✳. With yoga as a vehicle, each aspect of Self aspires toward harmony. As this balance develops, the various facets become integrated in relationship with one another, supporting your holistic development as both an individual and a rider, while enhancing your relationship with the horse.

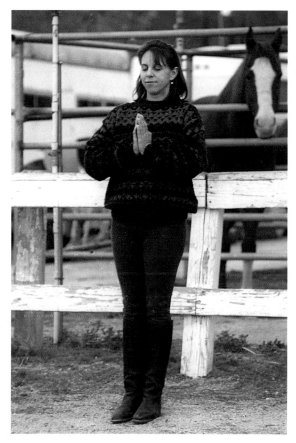

Prepare Your Body For Riding

In the same manner that basic dressage supples and balances the horse, preparing it for any riding task, yoga will supple and balance you as a rider, preparing your body to more successfully engage in any riding activity. Practicing yoga as a riding warm-up helps to counteract the effects of stress on your body, ensuring a more pleasurable ride by "de-stressing" you before you mount the horse.

Yoga practice guides you toward integration and wholeness.

Relaxing and Energizing

Almost everyone has areas of tension in their body, and equestrians are certainly no exception. The gentle, flexible nature of yoga is extremely effective in relaxing areas of the body that are tight due to stress. The positive effects of yoga include reducing tension, lowering blood pressure, and relaxing and soothing both body and mind, while increasing energy and mental clarity. Yoga encourages you to move slowly with awareness, helping tight areas to relax and stretch without force.

Body Awareness

Through yoga practice you can become better acquainted with your body and learn to be more physically "in" your body as opposed to living primarily in your intellect. Yoga for Equestrians enables you to develop increased body awareness both on and off the horse, furthering an understanding of how your body works. You will learn to better control and isolate the parts of your body and then operate your body more skillfully as an integrated whole. Improving awareness will assist you in maintaining the integrity of your riding position through all of the horse's gaits and transitions. Strengthening your body-mind connection by developing a heightened level of awareness will have a direct effect on your riding and your ability to influence the horse. As your awareness blossoms, you become better equipped to communicate with the horse, fostering a more productive alliance.

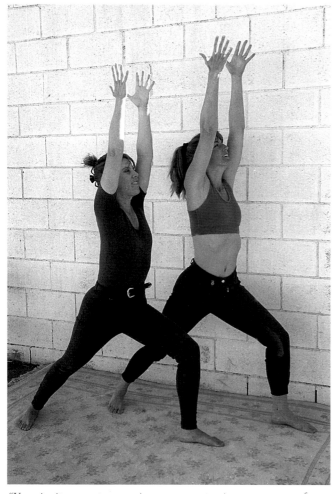

"Yoga invites you to move in new ways to give every part of you ... the gift of movement." [9] RACHEL SCHAFFER, *Yoga for Your Spiritual Muscles*

Improved Performance in the Horse

A direct result of integrating yoga with your riding will be a noticeable improvement in the horse's way of going. The horse will reflect the positive changes in your body-mind attained through yoga practice, demonstrating more willingness and cooperation in your work together.

Flexibility, Suppleness, and Tone

Yoga for Equestrians assists in developing the shock absorbing qualities of your joints—an important element in maintaining the integrity of your body alignment on the horse. Locked joints create blocks of tension in your body, preventing you from being able to absorb the horse's movement. Inflexible joints contribute to a loss of connection with the horse and instability in the saddle. Practicing yoga asanas will gently keep your joints lubricated and the surrounding muscles and ligaments supple, enabling you to develop greater flexibility in the saddle. Yoga for Equestrians also generates a more balanced tone in your large working muscle groups, important for stability and maintaining a secure position on the horse.

Alignment, Balance, and Poise

Consistent yoga practice can help correct asymmetries in your body and contribute to a more balanced alignment. By understanding the importance of an upright pelvis and aligned spine, you increase your ability to efficiently organize your body in a relaxed and balanced manner, both in and out of the saddle. Improving your physical posture through yoga practice will help you ride with more poise and grace.

Efficient Movement

A rider's balanced position in the saddle requires frequent adjustments. This dynamic process is improved by yoga practice, which teaches you to "use only what is needed." Yoga for Equestrians helps develop a body that is more efficient on the horse's back, fine-tuning your aids and eliminating excess physical movement. Your riding performance will reflect your increased awareness and body control.

Habits

Yoga for Equestrians can effectively help you become aware of your physical habits, then enable you to address them. As yoga practice brings your individual aspects into balance, you may notice that you are no longer at the mercy of your old, ingrained habits. Rather, you may be more in command of yourself in both body and mind. Yoga for Equestrians helps you to consciously respond to the events that occur throughout your day and in the saddle. Instead of reacting habitually, you will be able to choose the way you respond to any given situation.

In addition to improving your riding skills, the benefits of your yoga practice can carry over to your daily life activities, contributing to new, positive habits. You will discover that your practice can influence changes throughout your life, at home, work, school, or play, resulting in a better physical performance in all that you do, both in and out of the saddle.

"Yoga is introspective, allowing the practitioner to look within..." [10] JEAN COUCH, *The Runner's Yoga Book.*

Beyond the Physical

What distinguishes yoga from simple physical exercise is that it addresses you as a whole being. Because of its holistic nature, the benefits of yoga practice can reveal themselves on subtle levels, mentally, emotionally, and spiritually.

Yoga for Equestrians can...

• encourage you to participate fully in the moment, both on and off the horse;

• liberate the mind from unnecessary activity to better tune in to yourself and the horse;

• allow you to reverse escalating, out-of-control situations by returning your attention to the simplest common denominator: breathing;

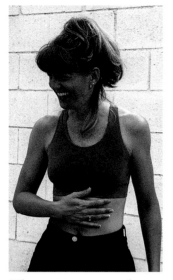

When we are open to what we are feeling, the feeling transforms and we find ourselves with greater energy and greater health." [11] ADELHEID OHLIG, *Luna Yoga*

"...the perceptive rider allows a mutually inclusive energy to flow between him/herself and the horse, staying in the moment, neither dwelling on the past nor anticipating the future." [13] SHERRY L. ACKERMAN, *Dressage in the Fourth Dimension*

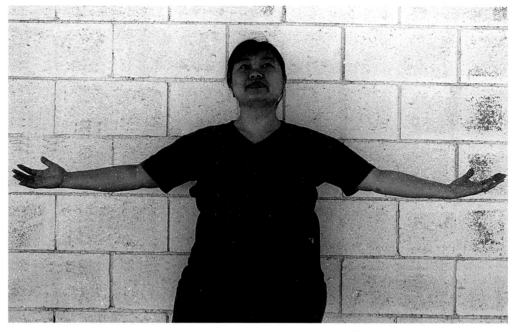

"Your spirit is the part of your being that allows for inner harmony." [12] JILL KEISER HASSLER, *Beyond the Mirrors*

- teach you to clear your mind, embrace silence, and better incorporate powerful meditation and visualization techniques into your riding repertoire;

- create a quiet mind, enabling you to achieve dynamic, rhythmic stillness on the horse;

- inspire you to observe your emotions objectively;

- encourage the *release*∗ of blocked emotions through the use of breathing and gentle movement, creating lightness and emotional health;

- nurture inner-harmony: an overall sense of well-being and peace of mind;

- increase sensitivity and develop intuition, both on and off the horse;

- encourage you to take responsibility for your own learning and development as a rider;

- foster an attitude of compassion and acceptance toward yourself and the horse.

CHAPTER THREE

Guidelines for Practice

I N THE SAME MANNER that equestrians commonly budget an hour or more for each lesson or ride, yoga practitioners ideally perform at least one full, uninterrupted practice of 60-90 minutes regularly, one or more times each week. Although achieving maximum results is directly related to the duration and regularity of your practice, the purpose of this book is to introduce yoga to you, the rider, in an easily accessible manner. As finding enough time to spend with your horse is often a challenge in itself, we focus on ways to integrate yoga into your riding repertoire in the most efficient and practical way possible.

There's no need to put off practicing Yoga for Equestrians until you have a sizable block of time—even a brief, regular practice can yield positive results in the performance of both horse and rider. Introducing yoga into your daily life can be as simple as practicing deep breathing in your car, a seated twist in your chair at work or school, or a forward bend while you're waiting for your tea kettle to boil. You can take ten minutes before you shower, five minutes before you tack up, or pick three of your favorite asanas to do as a cool-down after you ride. There are unlimited ways to bring Yoga for Equestrians into your daily routine. Get creative and start enjoying the benefits!

SECTION 1. Before You Begin

Before practicing Yoga for Equestrians, we recommend that you follow these guidelines to ensure your safety and enjoyment.

Safety

- Consult with your medical or health-care professional before you begin this program. If you are limited by a physical condition, prior injuries, or if you have any doubts about your capacity to perform yoga, you should obtain specific medical advice before beginning practice. Yoga for Equestrians is a gentle, safe form of exercise but not a substitute for medical treatment.

- Read through and understand this chapter before beginning. Read through each exercise before performing it and follow the sequence of steps for the asanas, pranayama, and awareness exercises.

- While doing the mounted exercises, we advise you to have an assistant available to attend to your horse. We also recommend wearing proper riding attire and protective headgear. Although some of the models in this book perform Yoga in the Saddle without a helmet, we strongly suggest that you wear one when mounted.

Nourishment

- Yoga should ideally be practiced on an empty stomach, so it is advisable to wait approximately two hours after a full meal and one hour after a light meal before practicing. If you need nourishment before yoga or riding, choose a light, healthy snack to boost your energy, such as a piece of fruit, granola or nutritional bar, juice smoothie, or something else of this nature.

- With every exhalation your body releases moisture. As breathing intensifies, moisture loss increases. It is important to remain hydrated by drinking enough water while riding and practicing yoga, especially outdoors and in warmer weather.

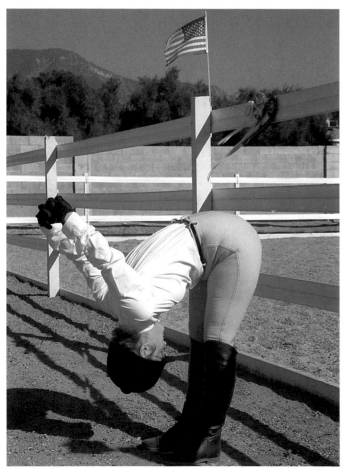

Yoga can be practiced anywhere!

Attire

- Yoga for Equestrians can be performed in regular riding attire such as breeches, jodhpurs or jeans—provided they do not drastically restrict movement. Otherwise, choose something tight and stretchy or loose-fitting.

- Your body should be kept warm while practicing. If you perform yoga outdoors in cool weather, take care to dress warmly from head to toe.

- Yoga is traditionally practiced barefoot to prevent slipping and to help you maintain a stronger sense of balance and stability. Yoga for Equestrians can easily be performed in riding boots; however, when feasible, we suggest that you practice barefoot.

Where to Practice

Yoga is an extremely adaptable activity, convenient to perform at home, work, school, and stable. You can further the development of your equitation skills even when not riding by practicing asanas and breathing techniques anywhere. Here are a few helpful ideas to allow you to take your practice with you, wherever you go:

- The optimal setting for yoga practice is a peaceful, quiet environment. However, realize that there will be times you are challenged by noise and distractions. At first, this may seem to present a problem, but it is not a reason to abandon your practice. Rather, see distractions as a wonderful opportunity to remain focused and calm while maintaining a conscious awareness of your surroundings. When noise and distractions intrude into your practice space and awareness, the following guidelines will help you to carry on under less than optimal conditions:

  - Gently draw your attention back to your breathing to help you remain focused on your practice.

  - Let normal barn noises simply become a tapestry of background sound.

  - Don't fight to erase distractions from your awareness, this only amplifies them. Rather, acknowledge them and let them flow past as you remain focused on the sound of your breath and the sensations of your body.

- Yoga for Equestrians can easily be performed at a horse show or competition; it requires no special equipment and can be done in show clothes. In the stable or at a show, it may not be comfortable for you to sit cross-legged for some of the seated asanas. Adapt these postures by using a chair, mounting block, or bale of hay instead.

- To provide extra cushioning for your practice, use a towel, exercise mat, Navajo, or horse blanket when practicing sitting and *supine*✶ poses indoors or out.

SECTION 2. Enhancing Your Practice

Beyond mere exercise, Yoga for Equestrians is multifaceted, engaging body, mind, and spirit. Following are some key thoughts to consider while practicing. Applying these ideas will enable you to glean the most from your time and make your yoga practice more rewarding and enjoyable.

Beginner's Mind

When enthusiastically approaching a task for the first time, the student's mind tends to be more open and receptive to new information. For example, if you eagerly attend a clinic with a new trainer, it is to your advantage to suspend your usual way of doing things so that you may try the new techniques offered, becoming open to receive new learning experiences, which is why you are there in the first place. This open-minded approach is often referred to as *beginner's mind*✶: a state of mental receptivity, as if you were an "empty cup" ready to be filled with new knowledge and learning. In this state of mind, you are able to approach any situation as if it were brand new, setting aside predetermined expectations in order to see clearly what is before you. If you are full of your own criticisms, ideas, and opinions, there will be no room for new observations and physical possibilities—you must first create space in order to receive.

As you approach both yoga practice and riding, make every effort to do so with a beginner's mind. With your mind open and judgment set aside, you are receptive to the

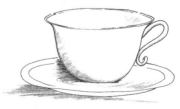

Let your mind be like an empty cup, ready to be filled with new information.

subtle feedback of your own body and that of the horse, making room for greater possibility and advancement. Remember, in yoga practice, riding lessons, clinics, or new training situations, what your mind knows in theory, your body requires time and progressive training to incorporate.

Allowing

In yoga, there is no forcing but rather steady encouragement to let go of the common inclination to "do too much" or "try too hard." The "no pain, no gain" mentality so often advocated by more rigorous exercise programs has never been part of yoga. The gentle practice of Yoga for Equestrians encourages you to listen to your body as you perform smooth, fluid movements, then hold a steady pose, releasing all unnecessary muscular tension.

Yoga is about allowing. Instead of forcing or pulling yourself into an asana, allow your body to open gently into the pose. You may even feel as though you are "melting" into the asana as you allow gravity and your breath to assist your body to find its place in the pose.

Breathing

Remember to *breathe deeply* throughout all the asanas as you practice. Proper breathing (discussed in detail in Chapter 4) keeps you focused in the present, improves your concentration, and enhances fluidity and grace in your movements. Throughout this book, you will be reminded that breathing is fundamental to both yoga practice and riding.

The correct use of your breath is invaluable in preventing excessive muscular strain. As you come into an asana, imagine that you can "breathe yourself into the pose" and allow your body to find its own comfortable place within the asana. During rhythmical asanas, imagine your breath literally "fueling" your movements and encouraging them to become more natural, fluid, and intuitive. While practicing yoga, let your breath lead and see where it takes you!

Finding Your Edges

In yoga practice, perform the asanas with slow, fluid movements, remaining aware of your *edges*✻—the fine line between working a bit more intensely and pushing beyond your limitations. There are no violent or abrupt movements in yoga, rather, you are encouraged to move deliberately with awareness. With each breath, strive to remain in the present. Listen to your body's feedback as you feel for your edges, to help prevent injury. Your body has ample time to communicate as you create the space to listen. Your edge can change from one day to the next and sometimes from one breath to the next. Your edge may alert you to pull back slightly or that it is time to move a little deeper. By listening to your body closely, you can learn to let go of harsh expectations and self-judgments, responding with enhanced clarity and objectivity. Learning to listen in this way during your yoga practice will enable you to take this sensitivity to your riding, as you tune in to both yourself and the horse with increased awareness.

"The body has edges that mark its limits in stretch, strength, endurance, and balance...This edge has a feeling of intensity, and is right before pain, but it is not pain itself."[14] JOEL KRAMER, *Yoga Journal*

Sun - Moon

As you discover your edges you will begin to notice the polarities within yourself—masculine/feminine, sun/moon, advance/yield, dark/light. Feel the ongoing dance as you advance into each pose, then allow your body to yield within the pose, dynamically balancing these polarities. As you perform the asanas, you develop a sense of inner harmony as a result of the increased balance between your "Sun" qualities and "Moon" qualities. Working with this inner balance will greatly improve your riding and is a gift you take with you to the horse (for more on polarities, see "Riding Without Force" in Chapter 5).

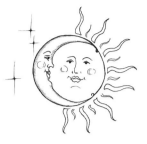

Balancing your "Sun" qualities and "Moon" qualities fosters an inner harmony – a gift to take with you to the horse.

Balancing Your Practice

Once you have become familiar with Yoga for Equestrians and are comfortable practicing the asanas and pranayama, you may choose to customize the existing sequences to suit your individual needs. In tailoring your own practice, it is important to bear in mind one of the fundamental concepts of yoga: *balance*. Balancing your practice begins with your selection of asanas. For example, if your goal is to build strength and tone in your abdominal area through specific asanas, be sure not to neglect the rest of your body. Incorporating a variety of asanas into your practice will enable you to develop an overall balance of muscular strength, tone, and flexibility.

Another way to maintain balance in your yoga practice is by using *counter-poses*✳. A counter-pose is an asana that provides a complementary, opposing movement to another. For example, if you have just completed a backbending pose, doing a forward bend will balance your back by moving it in the opposite direction. Throughout the book we offer counter-poses after specific asanas wherever applicable.

In your yoga practice, your body may welcome some of the asanas readily, while others seem impossible. Rather than avoiding the asanas that seem difficult and selecting only the ones you can perform easily, we encourage you to see the challenging poses as an opportunity to create balance in your practice. Consciously exploring the more challenging poses will enable you to gradually go beyond limitations in both mind and body to discover what you are capable of. Just as the horse's work ideally involves a variety of physical and mental challenges, incorporating progressive levels of difficulty that teach him to work through resistance and expand the boundaries of what is comfortable, we encourage you to do the same with your yoga.

Emotions

Deep-seated feelings that are not acknowledged or released can become lodged in different areas of your body and manifest as *dis-ease*: chronic tension, discomfort, minor aches, pain, or illness. As you move through your yoga practice stretching new areas of your body, you may experience the physical release of an emotion you have subconsciously stored in your body. This can often appear as spontaneous crying, a rush of anger or sadness, or a sudden experience of fear. Should you experience emotional release during or after your yoga practice (sometimes even a day or two later), use your breath to gently draw these emotions out. Allow yourself the freedom to experience your emotions without judgment and without trying to push them back below the surface.

Pain

Our modern culture considers pain something to avoid at all costs. Drugs and medications are overabundant and easily available. Unfortunately, these quick fixes only treat your symptoms and disguise the pain. This often leaves the true source of pain unresolved and likely to recur.

When approached constructively, pain and discomfort can be valuable teachers. If you experience pain or discomfort, stop and listen. What is this physical sensation communicating to you? Could it be that you have pushed too far past your edges? If so, what prompted you to do this? Do you detect a mental resistance or blocked emotion, such as fear, somewhere in your body? What is your experience of pain or discomfort saying to you? Listen closely, respect the information you receive, and respond appropriately. When you pay attention, pain can deepen the understanding of your yoga practice, your riding, and your Self.

Adapting for Health Concerns

We include gentle directions for progressing safely through each of the asanas in the Yoga for Equestrians program. However, we offer the following general guidelines for common injuries and conditions to enable you to get maximum benefit from yoga practice. Again, this is not a substitute for medical advice, and we recommend that you check with your health care practitioner for advice regarding your specific condition before beginning this program.

INVERTED ASANAS

Inverted poses involve being partially or totally upside-down. Although we have not included any full inversions in this book, we have included partial inversions. The following cautions may apply to any asanas where your head and upper body are upside-down. We suggest that you do not practice these poses if you have high blood pressure, or heart, retinal, or neck problems. If you feel particularly over-taxed or excessively hot after your ride, you may want to avoid doing inversions until you have normalized. Also, women are generally advised not to perform inverted asanas during pregnancy or menstruation.

MIGRAINE HEADACHES

If you are experiencing a headache or are especially prone to migraines, avoid practicing inverted or semi-inverted postures, which increase blood flow to the head. If your headache symptoms are minor and your health care practitioner is not opposed, exercise caution when performing these asanas, lowering and raising your upper body slowly, with awareness.

DISCOMFORT

Although moments of slight discomfort can be healthy signs of exploring your physical and mental limitations, you should never feel excessively uncomfortable while practicing yoga. If you ever feel dizzy, light-headed, out of breath, or fatigued, it is probably an indication that you are pushing farther than your body or mind is ready to go. If you experience any of these sensations, either lessen the degree of intensity within the pose or move slowly into one of the relaxation poses described later in this chapter.

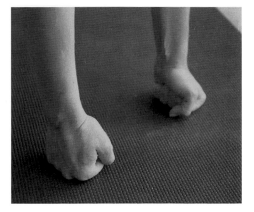

Wrist variation.

BACK INJURY

When coming up from any standing forward bend, you can protect your lower back by bending your knees. Use awareness when arching or bending backward. If these movements cause you back pain, avoid them. While practicing any twisting or backbending motion, it is imperative that you create length and extension through your spine. When lying on the floor, it is important to minimize the arch of your lumbar spine by keeping your lower back in contact with the floor. Placing a rolled towel under your knees or your hands underneath your sacrum can provide additional support.

NECK INJURY

Avoid tipping your head sharply back as this can compact the cervical vertebrae. Remember, your neck is part of your spine and you should always move with this in mind, both in and out of the saddle. For example, when twisting through your torso, do not turn your head severely over your shoulder, but allow your neck and head to follow the gentle rotation of your spine.

CARPAL TUNNEL SYNDROME∗ OR WRIST INJURY

With weight-bearing asanas, you can "stack" your wrists in a fist instead of using flat hands to support your body. This will prevent strain to your wrists and eliminate the possibility of over-bending. (See photo above.)

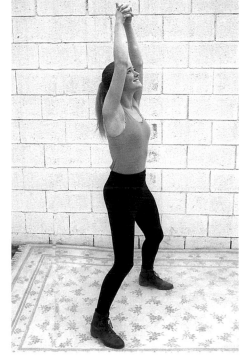

KNEE INJURY

Strengthening the quadricep (upper thigh) muscles will generally help protect your knees from strain. In addition, it is important to keep your knee and shin in vertical alignment. Avoid twisting your legs, hips, or feet in any way that would force your knees out of alignment with your lower leg. Proper alignment will help prevent strain or injury to the knee.

Enjoyment

Above all, do what feels good and allow your practice to be fun and enjoyable. Yoga is a treat for your body! When you think, "I can spend time doing something that feels good to my body" rather than "I *have* to do my exercises now," you will have a lot more fun. It's not often you hear someone say "Oh *darn*, I have to eat dessert again!"[16] Get the idea?!

Have fun with yoga!

Relaxation

"Relaxing involves the whole person. There is no point in having a relaxed body if your mind still races at sixty miles per hour. Similarly, it is of little use to have a calm, peaceful mind if the body is tense and tight. Body and mind affect each other. When one is calm and centered, the other can follow more easily."[17] RACHEL SCHAFFER, *Yoga for Your Spiritual Muscles*

It is traditional in yoga to finish all practices with a "final relaxation," providing an opportunity for your body to assimilate the energy that you have generated during your practice and put it to good use. A final relaxation allows your body, mind, and spirit to get the most from your practice, even if it is short. Relaxation will also help you feel renewed and refreshed. It is a time to bask in the sensations of your practice. This is also a good opportunity to offer gratitude to your body for all that it does for you. For the practices outlined in this book, approximately two to five minutes of final relaxation is appropriate, although you can certainly rest longer if you wish.

Following yoga practice, there are several ways for you to relax. A Deep Relaxation in Corpse Pose is the most advantageous, although not always feasible if you do not have a place to lie down comfortably. The asanas for a Medium Relaxation and a Light Relaxation allow you to benefit from this important phase of any yoga practice, anywhere.

CORPSE POSE

DEEP RELAXATION

RIDER BENEFITS: The deepest level of relaxation and rejuvenation is induced by Corpse Pose, the traditional pose for finishing a yoga practice. It is done laying on your back and should follow a cool-down practice, when you can allow yourself deep and complete relaxation. Corpse Pose is often referred to as Final Relaxation or Deep Relaxation Pose, the classic yoga position for inducing a deep and peaceful state throughout the body after a practice. Use Corpse Pose after any yoga practice to bring complete and total relaxation to your body and mind. Many students jokingly refer to this as their favorite yoga asana!

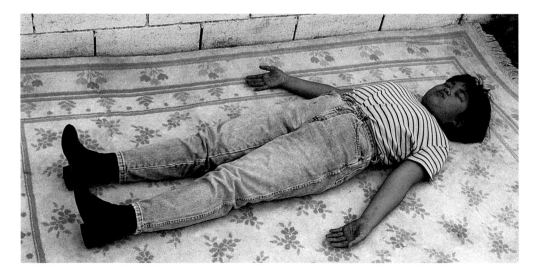

Corpse Pose.

TIP: Once in Corpse Pose, you should remain there for at least 5 minutes, more if you can, to gain the full benefit. If you experience any discomfort in your lower back, you can place a rolled towel, or the like, under your knees to reduce tension.

1. Lay flat on your back with your feet about shoulder width apart and your arms slightly away from your body, palms up. Draw your shoulders down away from your ears and lengthen the back of your neck. Relax your lower back and legs.

2. When comfortable, start consciously relaxing each area of your body, beginning with your feet and legs, working your way gradually through your hips, back, abdomen, chest, shoulders, arms, neck, face and, finally, your mind. Take as much time as you need. Once you have relaxed your whole body, simply let go of all effort and allow yourself to be still. Relax for 5-10 minutes, varying the time as it feels appropriate.

3. Come out of Corpse Pose slowly and gradually. Begin to bring your awareness back to your body by deepening your breath, then gradually stretching your body, letting it wake up at its own pace. Sit up slowly and take a few deep, relaxing breaths before moving on.

CHILD'S POSE

MEDIUM RELAXATION

RIDER BENEFITS: For a medium level of relaxation after practice, try Child's Pose. This asana provides an effective, restful release for your body as a final relaxation and is perfectly suited for a cool-down practice, as well. Child's Pose is a very relaxing and rejuvenating resting pose. This gentle inversion releases the lower back and shoulders and increases blood flow to the brain.

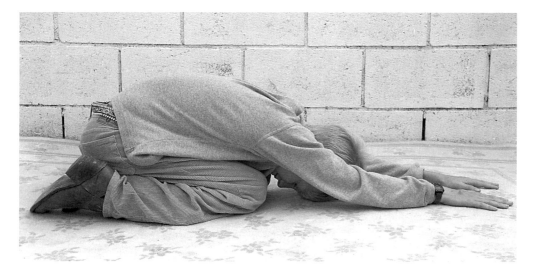

Child's Pose.

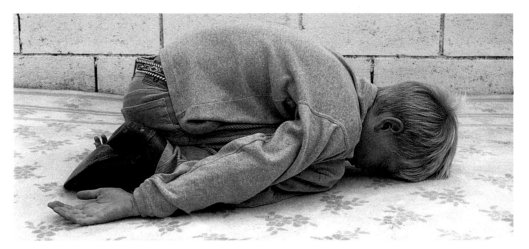

Child's Pose Variation.

TIP: Use this pose at any point during your practice should you feel weary or fatigued. Child's Pose is also a good transition from one asana to the next when practicing supine and sitting poses. If you perform Child's Pose before riding as part of your warm-up, follow with the Light Relaxation in Easy Pose to make sure that you are alert.

1. Kneel down and sit on your heels with the tops of your feet flat on the floor. Spread your knees wide enough apart to give your torso room to rest between them.

2. Walk both hands forward as you lower your upper body. Stretch your arms out in front of you and rest your forehead on the floor.

3. Breathe deeply and rest, allowing all your tension to flow out into the ground with each exhalation. With each inhalation, draw in rejuvenating energy from the earth. Stay here for at least 8 deep breaths.

4. Slowly walk your hands toward your body, gradually coming back to your starting pose. Focus your attention inward and breathe deeply before moving on.

VARIATION: Bring your arms to lie relaxed against your sides. Try both positions of Child's Pose to see which you prefer.

EASY POSE

LIGHT RELAXATION

RIDER BENEFITS: A light level of relaxation is most suitable for the transition between a riding warm-up and mounting, allowing you to remain sharp and alert for your subsequent work on the horse. Light relaxation is best achieved in Easy Pose. You will probably recognize Easy Pose as the simple cross-legged sitting position you learned as a youngster. Easy Pose also provides a stable and balanced base from which to perform seated asanas or to rest and meditate.

TIP: If you experience tension in your back or if you are rounding your back in this pose, elevate your seat bones slightly by sitting on a pillow, rolled towel, or saddle pad.

1. Bring one foot in to rest against the opposite inner thigh, then cross your other leg in front, tucking that foot under your other knee. It is good to get into the practice of switching legs on a regular basis to keep your body balanced.

2. Breathe deeply into your abdomen and feel your seat bones in contact with the floor. Imagine them sinking downward. Holding this sensation, allow your spine to extend upward as you sit erect and relaxed.

3. Sit quietly with your eyes closed. Take at least 8 deep, slow, and rhythmic breaths, and bring your awareness inward.

4. Follow with a moment of stillness as you continue to focus inward before opening your eyes and completing this Light Relaxation.

VARIATION: Sitting variations can be performed in a chair, on a mounting block, or bale of hay. If you are on the move, such as at a show or competition, relaxation can be also achieved while standing in Mountain (p. 71).

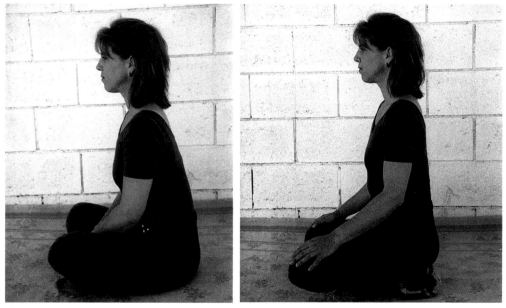

Easy Pose.   *Easy Pose Variation.*

PART II

The Foundations of Union

"The union between horse and rider is a sacred sacrifice where each learns to treat the other with the utmost respect and reverence. The rider throws away cruel training tools and brings compassion to the work. The horse gives up its vices and gains confidence in, and respect for, the process."[18]

SHERRY L. ACKERMAN, *Dressage in the Fourth Dimension*

✦

CHAPTER FOUR

The Art of Breathing

YOUR BREATH has the potential to deepen your connection with the horse. Correct breathing creates relaxation in both body and mind, enabling you to focus and maintain your balance and rhythm while riding. Breathing deeply and rhythmically infuses movement with greater fluidity and grace and, when you breathe fully, you allow freedom of movement in the horse by first creating freedom in your own body.

In contrast, when you hold your breath, such as during times of deep concentration or anticipation, movement becomes mechanical as your body locks up, arresting the flow of energy. Learning how to breathe correctly and to tap into the power of your breath will have many positive effects on your riding.

SECTION 1. The Bridge Between Body, Mind, and Horse

The natural and apparently simple act of breathing is a great connecting force between our body, mind, and spirit. It is something that our body does *unconsciously*, yet we can also control it with our *conscious* mind. For this reason, yoga teachings consider the breath to be a bridge between all our aspects. For equestrians, the breath can also bridge the gap between rider and horse.

Prana and Pranayama

Breath gives life and energy to the body. On a physical level, it nourishes the body, bringing in life-giving oxygen and then releasing impurities and carbon dioxide. To many, this describes the entire extent of the breath's capability. However, in yoga and many other ancient teachings and cultures, the breath has long been considered to have a profound effect at multiple levels. Donna Farhi, in *The Breathing Book*, shares some ancient translations for the word "breath" that explore its archetypal meanings. For example, "*In Greek*, psyche pneuma *meant breath/soul/air/spirit. In Latin,* anima spiritus, *breath/soul. In Japanese,* ki, *air/spirit; and in Sanskrit,* prana *connoted a resonant life force...In Chinese the character for 'breath'* (hsi) *is made up of three characters that mean 'of the conscious self or heart.' The breath was seen as a force that ran through mind, body, and spirit like a river running through a dry valley giving sustenance to everything in its course.*"[21]

In yoga, the breath is considered the physical manifestation of our energy or life-force, known as *prana*∗. This energy imbues us with life and vitality, animating all our movements. Prana is also understood as a universal force, present in every living thing and even in the air we breathe, always available if we are open to receive it. In Yoga Journal's *Yoga Basics*, Mara Carrico explains that in the Western world, energy is viewed as "*finite and measurable, something we constantly need to replenish.*" However, in Eastern thought, "*Energy or Prana...is everywhere and in limitless supply—all we have to do is open ourselves up as vehicles or channels for this omnipotent and omnipresent force.*"[22] It is largely through the use of the breath that we are able to do this.

Early yoga practitioners found it was possible to consciously become calm and focused, or energized and empowered, simply by using different methods of breathing. In the practice of yoga, these methods are known as pranayama. *Prana*, which translates as life-force, combined with *yama*, meaning control, can be interpreted as control over the flow of life-force moving through you. Pranayama are techniques or exercises that make a natural, unconscious process conscious. But pranayama do not involve "over-controlling" in a manner that becomes restrictive. Instead, these techniques provide a way to liberate the breath in order to reawaken aspects of the body-mind that have been neglected or forgotten.

Use the pranayama in this book as guides to help you discover and learn about your own unique breath. Like the asanas, they are not goals in and of themselves, but tools for learning more about yourself as you journey toward Union with the horse.

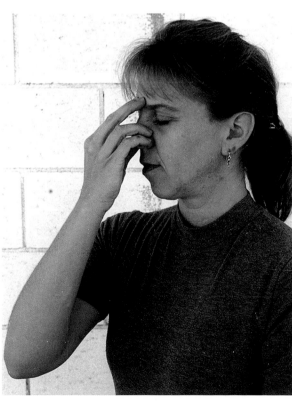

Alternate Nostril Breath.

ALTERNATE NOSTRIL BREATH

RIDER BENEFITS: An excellent pranayama for riders, the Alternate Nostril Breath relieves anxiety and creates a sense of calm, promoting the emotional stability essential for riding. Ideal to include in a general rider warm-up or before going into the show ring. This fundamental yogic breathing exercise will deepen the rider's breath and assist in balancing, centering, and focusing the mind.

TIP: To fully understand the sequence, read through all of the steps before beginning this pranayama.

1. Sit comfortably in Easy Pose, on a chair, mounting block, or bale of hay. Stretch up tall through your spine and breathe normally.

2. Using your right hand, rest your thumb lightly on the right side of your nose, your forefinger and middle finger lightly between your eyebrows, and ring and pinkie finger lightly on the left side of your nose.

3. Close your right nostril with your right thumb, inhale deeply into your abdomen through your left nostril to a count of 8. Keeping your right nostril closed, also close the left nostril with your ring and pinkie fingers, and hold your breath for a count of 8. Release only your thumb and exhale completely through your right nostril to a count of 8, drawing your abdomen in and up as you push all the air out.

4. With your left nostril still closed, and without pausing, inhale deeply through your right nostril to a count of 8. Close your right nostril and hold for a count of 8. Then release your left nostril and exhale fully for a count of 8. This completes one full cycle of Alternate Nostril Breath. The steps are clarified as follows:

> Inhale, left nostril 8 counts
>
> Hold inhalation 8 counts (both nostrils closed)
>
> Exhale, right nostril 8 counts
>
> Inhale, right nostril 8 counts
>
> Hold inhalation 8 counts (both nostrils closed)
>
> Exhale, left nostril 8 counts

5. Repeat at least 3 more times, completing 4 full cycles in all. As this breath becomes easier for you, you can increase the number of cycles as you desire.

Energy Flow

Have you ever noticed, while at a horse show perhaps, several competitors riding the same class, pattern, or course, all performing well from a technical standpoint, yet one pair stands out from the rest; they have that certain "something?" What you noticed was the dynamic expression of energy. The special horse and rider pair that caught your eye were animated from the inside, charged with life-energy. Prana was flowing through both horse and rider without any hindrance or blocks, each partner able to include the other in their flow.

This is the quality that "brings them to life" before your eyes. This exchange of energy can elevate riding performance to an art. When a rider learns to foster this energy flow within herself, she can then include the horse in that flow, creating a bridge and deepening the level of communication in the partnership.

Often, energy gets "stuck" in different areas of the body, limiting freedom of movement. For example, if you are habitually tense or stressed, you hold your body tight, closing certain areas off to the flow of prana and creating an *energy block*✱. An energy block is any area in your body that is not fluid and animated, but full of resistance, inhibiting the flow of prana.

A specific type of energy block can result from a past injury, such as damage to the shoulders, knees, or back. Whether or not you still experience discomfort in that area, often your body remembers the original pain and will unconsciously continue to protect the area long after the injury has healed by restricting activity there, over-compensating with other parts of the body. The restriction of movement in these areas restricts the flow of prana, thus perpetuating the cycle.

Typical physical habits of your daily life can also contribute to inhibited energy flow through the body. Tasks such as sitting at a desk all day and not using your legs, or standing for long periods and never stretching your back, can cause you to "shut off" those parts of your body, making them seem numb or, quite literally, "life-less."

Learning to "breathe through your whole body" creates greater energy flow, bringing more vitality and fluidity to your movements both on and off the horse. This helps to release energy blocks in areas of your body where prana is not freely flowing. Using your breath to bring life to these blocks, you can gently allow these areas to move fluidly and in concert with your body as a whole. When your body moves freely, uninhibited by energy blocks, your riding will reflect suppleness and harmony, resonating with the horse, infusing your horse-rider partnership with expressiveness and brilliance.

Directing the Breath

With a complete understanding of your body's breathing mechanism, enhanced by the creative use of your conscious mind, you can direct your breath deep into your abdomen, through each of your limbs, along your spine, and even to the tips of your fingers, toes, and ears! It is possible to feel the energy and lightness created by your breath as it travels to each part of your body and infuses every cell. Wherever you direct your breath, your awareness travels with it, thus establishing a close connection between body and mind.

"The act of release frees you from tightness, tension, or grasping."[23] CATHERINE PONDER, *Open Your Mind to Receive*

When your breath is limited, either physically or energetically, your capacity to bring this full flood of energy and life-force to your whole body is diminished. If you are accustomed to breathing shallowly, it may feel awkward, even strenuous, to deepen your breath with increased involvement of your abdominal muscles. However, as with all facets of yoga, a little practice will yield gratifying results and allow you to gradually increase your ability to deepen and guide your breath.

Breathing into a particular area of your body places that area foremost in your attention. A rider can use this effective technique to address specific areas of the body that may feel blocked, rigid, or resistant. It is possible to breathe energy and vitality into those areas, improving the relaxation and suppleness of the body. For example, perhaps the area surrounding each of your hip joints is especially tight, causing you to ride with poor leg contact and a braced seat. Targeting deep, rhythmic, relaxing breaths into this blocked area will encourage more release and openness. (In Chapter 5, you will find additional techniques for clearing energy blocks).

This gentle approach coaxes your body to release while you maintain a state of relaxed concentration, as opposed to commanding or forcing the change. It is more effective to use the breath as a tool directed toward releasing energy blocks and tension in your body, and to assist in attaining the ultimate goal of releasing with relaxation.

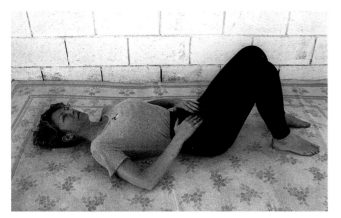

Complete Breath.

COMPLETE BREATH

RIDER BENEFITS: The Complete Breath demonstrates how the body was designed to breathe. Drawing the breath deep into the torso through three distinct areas, the rider's lungs expand fully as the muscles involved in the breathing process engage. The Complete Breath teaches the rider to direct the breath with increased awareness. This pranayama provides a tool for the rider to use in lowering her center of gravity in any mounted or unmounted activity.

1. Begin lying down with your knees bent, feet flat on the floor. Place your palms on your abdomen just below your navel. Imagine your hands possessing a magnetic pull that helps direct your breath deeper into your abdomen. With a long, gradual inhalation, draw your breath down into your abdomen and feel it expanding beneath your hands. Now, feel your rib cage expand fully, sideways, forward, and back, followed by your upper chest swelling with your breath. Allow this Complete Breath to fill your lungs to their fullest capacity. Pause before exhaling to experience the fullness and presence of your breath.

2. Exhale, and reverse the process by first contracting your abdominal muscles as you draw them toward the floor. They will "sink" down as you begin pushing the air outward, assisted by your hands. Feel the exhaled air pass through your rib cage. As the muscles between your ribs contract, your rib cage will begin to constrict, pushing the air higher up through your body. Continue to empty your lungs and expel air though your upper chest, which sinks down toward the floor. Pause and experience the absence of your breath before inhaling.

3. Continue the Complete Breath several times, spending a few moments breathing fully. Direct your breath through these three levels—abdomen, rib cage, and upper chest—on each inhalation and exhalation. Remain aware of your hands on your abdomen, rising and falling with each breath. Breathing this deeply may feel unnatural at first; most people are not accustomed to breathing this consciously. Stay with it until you begin to feel the entire breathing process becoming rhythmical and fluid. Rest and breathe normally.

VARIATION: Try performing the Complete Breath sitting and standing.

SECTION 2. Breathing and Riding

How you breathe may very well mirror how you ride and thus how your horse performs. Examine the correlation between your breathing patterns and your typical ride. If your breathing is shallow and concentrated in your upper chest, you will likely experience a "shallow" connection with the horse, feeling as though you are hovering in the saddle, rather than feeling plugged in. Rapid or hurried breathing can affect rhythm, resulting in abrupt or erratic movements in the saddle, contributing to nervousness in a horse who may tend to rush or spook. Breathing that lacks vitality may result in your dulled responses and lazy movement, increasing the possibility of riding mishaps and eliciting lackluster qualities in the horse. Or you may find yourself holding your breath, which causes you to tire easily, creates tension, and restricts freedom in both you and your horse.

In contrast, deep, rhythmic breathing while in the saddle increases your *aerobic*∗ endurance and communicates such qualities as regularity, relaxation, and focus to the horse, encouraging these same qualities in your equine partner. Just as constricted breathing creates tension and stiffness, deep, steady breathing creates rich, fluid movement and the rider's increased capacity to sustain physical activity on the horse. As you converse in the physical language of riding, your personal breathing style communicates a breadth of information you may not be conscious of. This is apparent because the horse reflects the rider so well, mirroring your use of body and breath.

Deep breathing creates movement all the way down to the muscles in your hips and pelvis, and each breath you take can be felt by the horse through your seat. He can feel your hips soften and widen, as well as the rhythm you create with your breath. As prana flows freely throughout your body, it can increase the mobility and flexibility of your back, arms, and legs as you ride, which the horse will sense and respond to. From your legs wrapped around his rib cage, the horse can detect subtle changes in the energy coursing through your lower body. If prana is restricted and your legs grip excessively, the horse will be tense and find it difficult to breathe under you. With sensitive leg contact, traditionally known as "the breathing leg," you can literally respond to the horse's inhalations and exhalations, and follow the movements of his barrel with your legs.

The horse often audibly exhales in rhythm with his movement. Listen to these sounds as you ride, and learn to incorporate the rhythm and sound into your own breathing patterns to deepen your connection with the horse. Often, administering sharp leg aids will cause the horse to expel his breath suddenly, as if he were being punched, interfering with his natural breathing rhythm. The goal then is *not* to interfere with the horse's natural breathing rhythm, but to become absorbed in it by coordinating your own breathing patterns with his. As riders, we find ourselves in the humble position of re-learning a process that our four-legged partners have never forgotten: to move in natural rhythm with the breath. A two-way dialogue develops as you gain the sensitivity to respond to your horse's breathing patterns as he responds to yours.

As you explore both the rhythm and depth of your breath, using it to direct prana through all areas of your body, be mindful of the ways that your body responds. As you master the use of your breath to direct prana through your own body, you can then learn to direct it through the horse.

Bringing more prana into the horse-rider partnership will create the desirable qualities you seek. For example, if the horse lacks expression and his movement is uninspired, try breathing more powerfully, deeply, and rhythmically in time with his strides. If the horse's *cadence*∗ is uneven or choppy, breathe with more definition and regularity. The

"Breathing is the expression of life...how we breathe is how we live."[24] *BIJA BENNETT, Breathing Into Life*

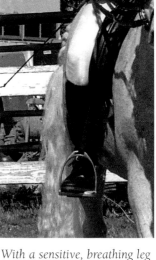

With a sensitive, breathing leg you can respond to the movement of the horse's body as he breathes.

horse will respond both mentally and physically to the improved steadiness and relaxation developed throughout your body. As you become better able to stabilize your own rhythm through the use of your breath, you will provide the horse with a dependable meter to follow while increasing your stamina in the saddle. We encourage you to use pranayama to rediscover the balancing characteristics of your own breath, letting it become a reliable bridge between you and every horse you ride.

If you have never considered the horse's breathing or have been unable to actually feel it, try the following simple mounted exercise to develop awareness of the horse's breath. Have someone read it aloud as you begin at the halt with an assistant holding the horse's head.

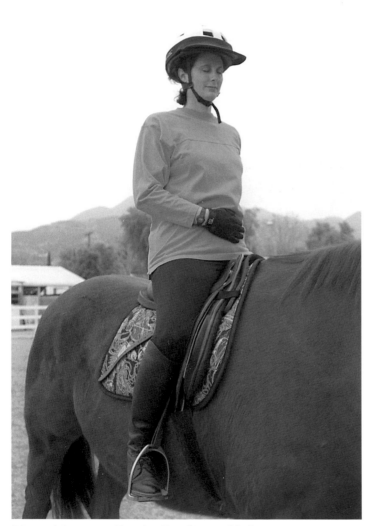

Mounted Awareness Exercise: Breathing and Riding.

MOUNTED AWARENESS EXERCISE:
Breathing and Riding

1. Close your eyes. Take a few deep breaths and allow your body to relax and release tension. Breathe in through your nose and out through your mouth, relaxing your face and jaw. Sit upright and relax your body, focusing on the sound and sensations of your breath. Breathe rhythmically and deeply for several repetitions.

2. Now, move your awareness to the horse's body. Pay close attention to the quality of his back under your seat. Notice if it is relaxed or tense. Be aware of the horse's breath and notice how his back rises and falls; feel his barrel expand then release sideways as he breathes. The horse may sigh heavily as he relaxes, his movements becoming more pronounced. Notice how your body responds.

3. Tune in to the horse's natural breathing rhythm, and count each breath to increase awareness of his pattern. Determine how the horse's breathing compares to your own. Now, breathe in the same rhythm with the horse and notice how you feel.

4. Open your eyes and take up your reins. Walk and maintain this same awareness of the horse's breath. With close attention, feel how his breath and movements are naturally linked. Match your breath to the rhythm of his walk.

5. Finish this exercise at the halt and close your eyes as your assistant attends to the horse. Practice listening and feeling; mingle the sound of the horse's breath with your own.

SECTION 3. Developing the Cadence of Your Breath

In our technological society, the body often becomes the neglected servant of intellect. Some people feel most comfortable "in their mind" and pay little heed to balancing normal physical patterns of activity and rest, immobility and movement. Subsequently, these people may be reluctant to relinquish control of their body, to "let go" and move spontaneously, intuitively, and freely. We can all certainly take a cue from our four-legged equine partners by learning to express ourselves more fully through our body. Moving in rhythm with the horse, easily and harmoniously, can become simple and natural once you become capable of orchestrating rhythm through the use of your breath.

In yoga practice, integrating breath with movement brings the asanas to life. Likewise, the fundamental connection between breath and movement will bring life to your riding. Uniting your breath with your own as well as the horse's movement can heighten the level of lightness, fluidity, and energy in your riding. Your riding will become yoga!

Rhythm links breathe with movement. If you believe you "have no rhythm," it is time to release that limitation! Every *body* has the capacity to learn to move rhythmically. Rhythm is inherent in your body, which naturally and autonomically sustains rhythms of its own.

Whether the horse is rushing or lagging behind, you must be able to establish the desired rhythm in both mind and body, communicating a steady *tempo*＊ to the horse through your seat. This is a paramount skill as you progressively learn to set, adjust, and maintain the desired rhythm in the horse at each gait. In order to develop an even, balanced cadence or rhythmic flow in the horse's movements, you must first be able to *feel* a regular tempo throughout your entire body, allowing yourself to move fluidly, in time, without hindrance.

The rhythmic asanas presented in the next section will enable you to put this important concept into practice. While performing these asanas, imagine your breath literally "fueling" your movements as you *fill* your movements with your breath. Begin by establishing a conscious awareness of the natural rhythm of your breath, *then let your movements follow*. This approach can be used throughout your yoga practice and in your riding. Master the art of breathing in rhythm with movement on the ground first to establish your own cadence of breath and fluidity of movement, then recreate this feeling in the saddle to develop the horse's cadence, enhancing the expression and grace of your horse-rider team.

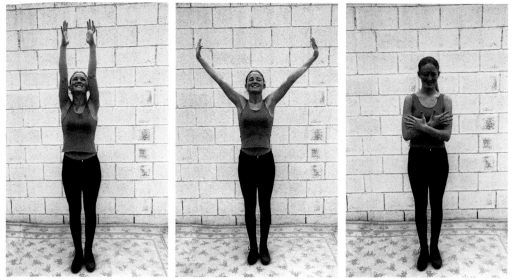

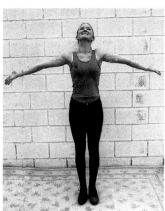

Arm Raise with Breath.

ARM RAISE WITH BREATH

- Look up past your fingertips
- Create a solid connection with the floor

RIDER BENEFITS: Introduces the rider to the use of the breath to initiate movement. Learning to move in rhythm with the breath creates fluidity and fullness in movement. Enhances a rider's self-awareness, expanding understanding of rhythm and cadence.

1. Stand with your feet together. Feel the soles of your feet in solid contact with the floor. Turn your attention inward as you allow your breath to become deep and fluid. Tune in to the natural rhythm of your breath. Close your eyes and listen until you can hear and feel your breath rising and falling rhythmically like ocean waves on the shore.

2. Maintaining awareness of your breathing pattern, on an inhalation, allow your arms to extend with your breath as they float out to your sides and up over your head.

3. As you exhale, let your arms follow your breath as they float down again. Continue to move your arms in concert with your breath, reaching up with each inhalation and floating them down with each exhalation.

4. Continue this fluid progression for at least 8 complete breaths. When you have finished, return to your starting pose and breathe normally.

WORK IN THE POSE: If you find that your arms begin to dictate the rhythm of your breath, shift your awareness and let your breath, once again, lead the movement. As you learn to fuel movement with your breath, you can increase the power of your breathing and bring more extension and energy to the motion of your arms.

VARIATION: Arm Raise with Breath can also be done while seated.

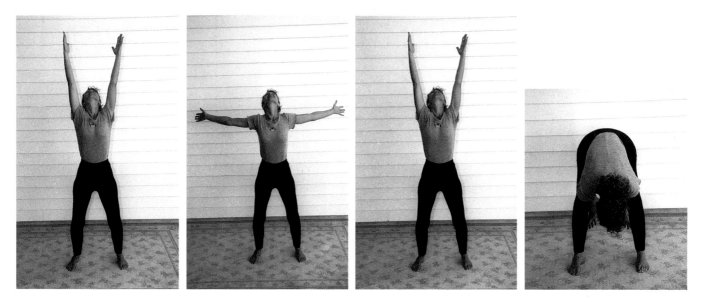

Breath of Joy.

BREATH OF JOY

- Open your chest to the sky
- Knees stay supple
- Put your heart into it!

RIDER BENEFITS: Invigorating, uplifting, and cleansing. It is an excellent way for the rider to release tensions of the day, rejuvenate, and energize before riding. This wonderful breath is expansive and liberating and, as the name implies, it tends to induce joy!

CAUTION: Horses tend to spook at this one, even at a distance, so be very aware and considerate of where you practice. For safety, keep well out of sight and reasonable earshot of any horses being handled on the ground or under saddle.

1. Stand with your feet together. Feel the soles of your feet in solid contact with the floor. Step your feet about shoulder width apart or wider. Keep your knees slightly bent and supple throughout the pose. You will inhale in three parts.

2. Inhale through your nose, filling your lungs about half way, as you swoop your arms straight overhead.

3. Inhale more as you swing your arms energetically out to each side.

4. Inhale even more as you swoop your arms overhead again.

5. With an exhilarating "Ha!," "Whoo!" or, at the least, an audible breath, swing your torso down, letting your arms make a full sweep down and back through your legs.

6. Without stopping, sweep your body right back up, going straight into the three-part inhalation and repeating the cycle again. Repeat this invigorating breath at least 4 times, working your way up to more repetitions as you get used to the increased intake of oxygen.

7. To finish, return to the starting position with your arms relaxed by your sides. Rest for a few breaths and enjoy the new sensations in your body.

RHYTHMIC SIDE STRETCH

- Keep knees elastic
- Back of neck is long
- Chest is open

RIDER BENEFITS: This rhythmic pose is excellent for helping the rider synchronize dynamic movement with the breath. It gives an invigorating stretch to the muscles along the sides of the torso, opens the chest, and loosens the arms and shoulders.

1. Stand with your feet together. Feel the soles of your feet in solid contact with the floor. Bend your knees slightly, keeping them soft and elastic throughout this asana. You will perform the following sequence of steps in one continuous, fluid movement.

2. As you inhale deeply, bring your fingertips together in front of your chest, palms down, and begin to stretch your right elbow up, your left elbow down. Look up as your right arm opens to extend straight up, stretching your right side as you reach straight down with your left arm. Gaze past your fingertips as you simultaneously incline your upper body to the left and sink a little deeper through your knees, bringing a greater stretch to the right side of your body. See that you don't fall forward

Rhythmic Side Stretch.

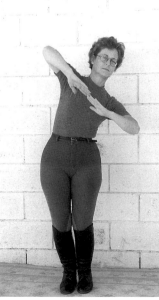

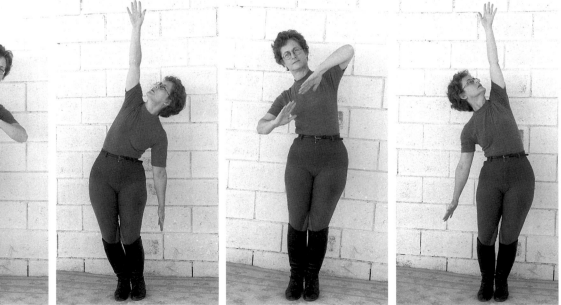

through your shoulders or hips.

3. As you exhale, sweep yourself back to your starting position, touching your finger-tips together in front of you, then repeat to the other side in one fluid movement.

4. Repeat this sequence, moving fluidly from side to side, following your breath, at least 8 times. When you have finished, return to your starting position; allow your arms to rest alongside your body and breathe normally.

WORK IN THE POSE: Energize your arms and torso with each inhalation, and contract your abdominal muscles with each exhalation.

CHAPTER FIVE

Exploring the Power
of Mind

YOUR MIND is one of the most miraculous and powerful gifts you have. In this chapter, we explore the power of your thoughts and how they influence your attitudes toward yourself, your riding abilities, and the horse. We examine how mental tools such as meditation, visualization, and *mantras*∗ are used in Yoga for Equestrians, providing positive, effective ways of facing common rider challenges like stress, scattered thinking, anxiety, and fear.

Learning positive mental habits that encourage "cleanliness" of mind can become as second nature as routine habits like brushing your teeth. Consciously washing out negative thinking and stilling your mind through visualization and meditation are invaluable to your yoga practice. These techniques encourage you to pay attention to your own inner dialogue and enable you to perceive the bigger picture: you and the horse as One.

SECTION 1. Creating with Thoughts

What you think about is what you create. Therefore, it is important to decide what kind of thoughts will exist in your mind. In her popular book, *That Winning Feeling*, author Jane Savoie describes the powerful abilities of the subconscious mind, which seeks to fulfill your predominant thoughts, either positive or negative. Savoie explains that the purpose of your subconscious *"...is to help you achieve your goal. It is like a guided missile. It gets a fix on its target—but if you shift your objective it will make whatever corrections are necessary to accomplish its mission."*[26]

Yoga for Equestrians encourages you to become more aware of your mental habits. Once your patterns have been examined and you have determined whether they serve or hinder your progress, we offer a selection of effective tools to help dispel fears, self-imposed limitations, and negativity from your thoughts. You can harness the power of your mind to *consciously* improve your effectiveness in the saddle and strengthen your partnership with the horse.

Facing Rider Challenges

A rider must learn to be attentive at all times in order to interpret the horse's signals. Establishing a mental connection with the horse can assist you in averting disaster or help you anticipate and prepare for the often abrupt movements and reactions of the unpredictable horse.

Being able to maintain a sense of calm while riding is a common challenge for most riders, especially in stressful situations when things can quickly escalate out of control. Regaining a sense of calm may seem nearly impossible, but it is feasible when you can still your mind. And, in facing most rider challenges, *that is exactly what you need to do.*

Perhaps you struggle with trying to focus and relax before a competition. Maybe certain riding situations trigger fear, which can make your ride less than pleasurable. Facing rider challenges begins by learning to clear and quiet your mind. Using the following strategies, you can consciously introduce new ways to react to stressful situations by choosing to think in a positive, encouraging manner, maintaining a sense of calm. These techniques, including meditation, visualization, and the repetition of a positive sound, word, or phrase known as a mantra, can help you consciously quiet your mind and refocus your responses during rider challenges. They will relax you, steady your emotions, and soothe your spirit. We encourage you to try all these methods and discover which ones really speak to you. When you find a technique that works well, remember to practice it often. You may discover that with practice, you can remain calm and relaxed even in the face of the most challenging situations in the saddle and out.

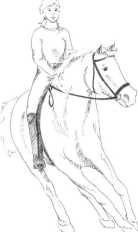

Facing a stressful situation begins by learning to clear and still your mind.

If you see things with a positive attitude, you can find a solution.[28] JILL KEISER HASSLER, *Beyond the Mirrors*

Relax Your Mind—Meditation

An unmonitored mind left to its own devices *"is by nature unsteady."*[29] Thoughts jump from one topic to the next, rushing out on tangents, never pausing, never resting. At its core, meditation is simply an effective means of stilling and clearing the mind; encouraging receptivity so that you are able to receive more subtle information. Meditation balances the mind, body, and spirit to create wholeness: a valuable asset for all equestrians.

Yoga for Equestrians teaches you how to integrate meditation into your riding repertoire, increasing mental stillness and nurturing the ability to reach this quiet state at will. Learning to become mentally relaxed and still through the practice of meditation elicits *"deep relaxation coupled with a wakeful and highly alert mental state."*[31] —the perfect mindset for the rider. Imagine the advantages of being able to quiet and focus your mind when facing the most challenging situations, including horse show jitters!

Through meditation, you can learn to quiet mental chatter, both on and off the horse, and remain fully present in each moment. You will find that when thoughts are suspended, your mind is quiet and open, with more room for new ideas and experiences. You may experience a sense of expansion, and increased ability to receive and process sensations and information. A quiet mind enhances your sensitivity and intuitiveness as a rider, heightening your ability to *listen* and respond to subtle feedback from both the horse and your expanded inner self.

"Ordinary experiences are limited by time, space, and the laws of causality, but the meditative state transcends all boundaries."[30] SIVANANDA YOGA VENDANTA CENTER, *Yoga Mind and Body*

How to Meditate

"Meditation means listening..."[32] ERICH SCHIFFMANN, *Yoga: The Spirit and Practice of Moving Into Stillness*

In his revolutionary book, *The Relaxation Response,* Dr. Herbert Benson describes the four elements necessary for meditation: a quiet environment, a comfortable position, an object of contemplation, and a passive attitude."[33] As you prepare to meditate, use the following guidelines to ensure that your meditation experience is both enjoyable and beneficial.

- *Quiet, peaceful environment*: Find a quiet place where you will not be disturbed. It is helpful to choose a space that you can use regularly.

- *Comfortable position:* Sit in a position that will be comfortable to hold for several minutes. You may prefer sitting in Easy Pose (perhaps with a cushion under your seat) or on a chair with a straight back. In the stable, you can sit on a hay bale, mounting block, or even the clean stable floor, with your back supported against a wall. Maintain an upright posture, keeping your spine straight.

- *Object of contemplation:* This can be almost anything. Try contemplating one of the following: the sound and rhythm of your breath; the repetition of a positive single-word mantra such as *relax, peace,* or *stillness*; or establish visual focus by looking intently at a candle flame or flower.

- *Passive attitude*: This is very similar to having a beginner's mind. Let go of expectations. Let go of trying. Do not become attached to the thoughts that travel through your mind or the sounds you hear. Acknowledge them, then let them go. Adopt an objective point of view. Allow and observe without judgment.

Below is an easy meditation that uses the sound of your breath to induce relaxation and stillness. Have someone read it for you, or record yourself reading this in a relaxed, soothing voice so that you can play it back as you meditate.

UNMOUNTED VISUALIZATION:
The Sound of Your Breath

Sit quietly and begin to breathe deeply. As you relax in both body and mind, let your breathing become regular and fluid. Slow your breathing tempo and notice the sound of your breath. Feel the ebb and flow as your breath washes through your body. Inhale through your nose and hear your breath like a wave gently rolling up to the shore. Relax your face and jaw as you exhale through your mouth. Hear your breath flowing out, like a wave returning to the sea. Simply experience the natural rhythm as you listen to the sound of your breathing.

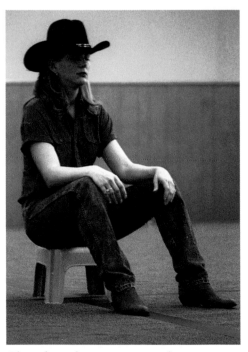

Through meditation, you can learn to quiet mental chatter and remain fully present in each moment.

If extraneous thoughts float into your mind, don't struggle with them—observe them without judgment. See these thoughts as clouds in the sky, drifting easily through your awareness. As you watch them gently float by, refocus your attention on the sound and feel of your breath. With each inhalation breathe in lightness and peace. With each exhalation, release thoughts or feelings that do not serve you.

Draw your attention deeply inward, and simply listen. Listen to the whispering voice, the voice of your heart, of your inner self. Let go of trying and just allow. Notice whatever comes to you. Feel this stillness within yourself and remember it. Know that you can come back to this feeling any time you wish.

To finish, wiggle your fingers and toes, slowly open your eyes, and stretch if you feel the need.

See Your Energy Flow—Visualization

Visualization is a technique that requires the conscious use of your imagination. Your imagination can become a tool to focus your goals and desires and provide the necessary energy to fulfill them. Shakti Gawain, author of *Creative Visualization*, explains, "*...you use your imagination to create a clear image of something you wish to manifest. Then you continue to focus on the idea or picture regularly, giving it positive energy until it becomes objective reality...in other words, until you actually achieve what you have been visualizing.*"[34] Yoga for Equestrians advocates visualization to assist you with both your practice and your riding: to develop a greater awareness of prana, the life-force energy in your body; to help clear energy blocks that impede your riding performance; and to incorporate the powerful technique of mentally rehearsing your ride before you mount up. Let's learn how to visualize!

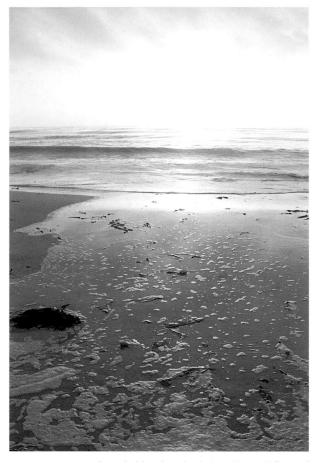

Experience your breath like the rhythmic ebb and flow of waves breaking on the shore. (Photo: Veronica Wirth)

How to Visualize

Visualization works best with your eyes closed and your attention turned inward. For some riders, painting a vivid picture in their mind's eye may not come easily. Don't be discouraged! For visualization to work for you, it is important to keep trying.

If you have trouble forming a mental picture, try using a "visual aid." With your eyes open, focus on an actual image, like a photo or sketch, or watch an accomplished horse-rider combination you admire. Gaze at your image, then close your eyes and try to recreate every detail in your mind. Keep trying until you recapture this image entirely in your imagination. You can also focus on the *idea* of what you would like to accomplish. Engage your emotions when visualizing. Adding *feeling* will activate your visualizations, producing energy to transform potential into reality. With practice, you can create detailed images in your mind of the desired changes you'd like to make, using visualization to help generate positive results.

To discover how visualization can help you achieve harmony in both your yoga practice and riding, try the following exercises. Have someone read to you or record yourself reading the exercises in a relaxed, soothing voice so that you can play them back as you visualize.

"Imagination is the ability to create an idea or mental picture in your mind."[35]
SHAKTI GAWAIN, *Creative Visualization*

Clearing Energy Blocks

This visualization enables you to *see* and *feel* the energy flow in your body and helps you learn how to work with it. In traditional yoga teachings, your physical body and the energy that animates it are inherently intertwined. Increasing your awareness of where life-force energy moves, or doesn't move, enables you to direct energy throughout your body where it is needed to create a balanced flow.

As discussed in Chapter 4, energy blocks occur in your body wherever the healthy flow of prana is inhibited. The following visualization will help you locate energy blocks. By imagining a bright colored light moving through you, you can learn to clear those blocks and revitalize your body.

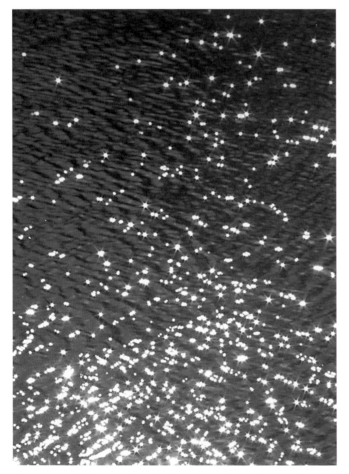

Imagine a bright sparkling light moving through you, clearing energy blocks and revitalizing your body.

UNMOUNTED VISUALIZATION:

Clearing Energy Blocks

Begin standing with your eyes closed, feet together, arms relaxed by your sides. Breathe deeply and relax. Bring your mind into a still, meditative state. Continue to breathe slowly and rhythmically.

Imagine you are standing in a sparkling pool of light; give it a color if you wish, one you can see vividly. As you stand in this pool, see and feel this bright light begin to travel upward through your body, starting at your feet. Let the light slowly wash up through you, cleansing and purifying you as it illuminates each part of your body. Feel yourself tingle and glow with this light.

As the energy travels through your body, notice if there are any areas where it feels stuck or has trouble moving through. These may be familiar as tight or tense places in your body. Breathe into those blocked areas. With your breath, direct the bright light gently and easily through. If you feel resistance, don't force the energy. Know that you are beginning a clearing process, and feel the energy healing your body.

Continue moving the light energy to the top of your head and out into the space above you. Bask in the glow. Feel your body revitalized, awake, and tingling with prana. Breathe deeply. Notice how you feel. To finish, wiggle your fingers and toes, slowly open your eyes, and stretch if you feel the need.

Lines of Energy

Yoga for Equestrian helps you visualize the flow of energy as it travels through the geometrical paths, or *lines of energy*★[36], produced in your body while performing the asanas (such as when both arms are extended, parallel to the ground). By seeing and feeling the lines of your body flowing with energy, you can increase the vitality of your practice, as well as your performance on the horse. You can consciously activate these lines during yoga practice to increase the flow of prana through your body, developing strength and endurance within each asana. This allows you to become more present and aware of your edges. Visualizing and directing prana along your lines of energy produces a natural and correct alignment within each posture and your position in the saddle.

The following visualization will guide you in feeling the lines of energy throughout your body as you direct energy purposefully along these pathways.

UNMOUNTED VISUALIZATION:
Lines of Energy

Begin standing with your eyes closed, feet together and arms relaxed at your sides. Breathe deeply and relax. Bring your mind into a still, meditative state. Continue to breathe slowly and rhythmically. Imagine a column of light emanating up from the ground under your feet. Give it a color if you wish, one you can see most vividly. See this pillar of light encircle your feet, climbing higher to encompass your legs. With each inhalation, draw this light up through your hips, torso, neck, and out the top of your head as it is carried on your breath. See and feel this column charged with prana extend straight through your body. Let the light strengthen and fortify you. Spend a moment experiencing this light; feel how invigorated you are!

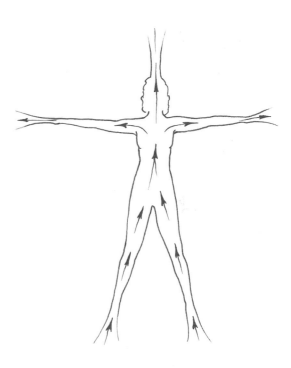

Next, step your feet about shoulder width apart. Imagine the vibrant column of light splitting into two streams that course through each of your legs, energizing them!

Slowly raise your arms straight out to your sides. Imagine the light dividing into two more columns that extend out through each of your arms. Feel the energy emanate outward through your fingertips. In this stance you create new pathways for the energy traveling through your body. Vividly imagine these pathways of bright light intensifying as your breath activates your lines of energy.

Now, gently open your eyes and continue to feel the lines of energy. If you begin to lose the sensation of the energy flow, you may wish to keep your eyes open only for a moment. With more practice, you can gradually keep them open for longer periods of time while experiencing your lines of energy. To finish, bring your arms back to your sides, wiggle your fingers and toes, slowly open your eyes and stretch if you feel the need.

By seeing and feeling the lines of your body flowing with energy, you can charge your practice, and your riding, with more vitality.

REFLECTIONS: *It is fun to experiment with this visualization by practicing it randomly throughout your day. For example, while standing in an elevator or waiting in line, recreate the column of light and extend it upward through your body. Feel it revitalizing you! As you clean, groom, or work with your hands, feel prana coursing through your extended arms and out your* *fingertips. Even as you sit at your desk, periodically check in with your body and imagine columns of light streaming through each leg, energizing them. Approach this exercise playfully— a lighthearted attitude will help you become accomplished at visualizing this column of light and activating your lines of energy at any time during the day.*

Mental Rehearsal of Your Ride

"Your ability to picture something that does not yet exist in your reality is one of your highest abilities."[37]
SANAYA ROMAN, *Spiritual Growth*

Have you ever thought, "I must remember to keep my heels down, my seat bones tucked under, my shoulders relaxed, my chest open, my eyes up, my hands still. Above all, I must not grip excessively with my knees!" Is this barrage of mental activity familiar? Analyzing and monitoring your every movement on the horse is not only difficult, but also potentially exhausting. The irony is that the effort involved in "working" on your position by manipulating parts of your body and focusing on separate tasks may cause you to lose sight of the *whole picture*. The Union you are seeking with your horse will continue to evade you. There is a better way to improve your riding.

The next exercise will help you create a visualization of a successful riding experience. Picture yourself and the horse in perfect alignment, moving together in balance; this image will clearly convey to your body-mind the situation you wish to create and communicate not only physical directions, but also *feelings*. Imagine what it *feels like* to ride this way, and your body-mind will do all it can to reflect your pictures back to you.

UNMOUNTED VISUALIZATION:
Mental Rehearsal of Your Ride

Find a comfortable place to sit down. Close your eyes and breathe deeply, slowly, and rhythmically. Bring your mind into a still, meditative state.

Now, create a picture in your mind's eye of the horse you will ride. See him as clearly as you can, in your favorite riding environment. Picture him in the tack you will use, with an alert, willing expression in his eye. See yourself on his back and vividly observe your riding attire. Notice the peaceful, happy expression on your face and experience these feelings as you continue breathing deeply.

Observe your body position on the horse at a halt. If you look tight or blocked anywhere, visualize yourself relaxing these areas. See yourself perfecting your position as you mentally scan your entire body, bringing it into a relaxed, balanced alignment. See yourself in a correct position in your mind and then *feel* how effortless it was to adjust your body.

Next, see yourself gather up the reins and begin your ride. Notice the fine quality of the horse's movement and how your body moves in harmony with his. Visualize each detail of your ride as you maintain a relaxed position, moving easily through every phase of your ride. Observe your transitions between gaits, and within gaits, and notice how the horse remains attentive to your aids. See your horse-rider team moving fluidly as One, communicating clearly to each other and enjoying this time together. Feel the satisfaction that comes from accomplishing your riding goals.

Spend time with this mental picture. Allow your body to remember the sensations of this imaginary ride and make them real. To finish, slowly open your eyes and stretch if you feel the need.

REFLECTIONS: *Practice this visualization regularly so that you can easily bring it to mind. Then, practice it before you mount up. For an added challenge, try this visualization with your eyes open. With this powerful visual ingrained firmly in your mind, your body will begin to make the necessary adjustments while you ride to correspond with your ideal picture and improve your performance on the horse. Try it!*

The Power of Words—Affirmations and Mantras

Although you may not always mean what you say literally (for example, "My back is *killing* me"), verbal language greatly influences your subconscious mind. Words are the audible representation of thoughts, ideas, and feelings. Becoming mindful of the power of words is an integral element in yoga and an important key to establishing Union.

Traditional yoga teaches that mantras can lead to powerful changes. A mantra—a sound, word, or phrase repeated over and over, as in a chant—is most often used in conjunction with meditation because the powerful tones of a mantra help focus the mind.

Focusing on a mantra can help *direct* your mind, allowing the extraneous thoughts to drift away, bringing your chosen idea to center stage. Using a mantra is a technique to consciously channel awareness. A mantra can be a single sound, tone, word, or phrase that captures either the feeling or idea you wish to focus on.

You can use your mantra anytime you wish to influence your state of mind, both in and out of the saddle. Choose an appropriate mantra, then repeat the sound, word, or phrase to yourself, silently or aloud. When repeating a key word or phrase that represents your riding goals, such as *Rhythm* or *Union*, you actively bring your mind's focus to this idea.

If you decide to use a series of words that form a statement, it is important to phrase this idea in a positive manner, affirming your statement to be true—even if it currently isn't. This type of mantra is called an *affirmation*, a powerful statement that is positive, spoken in the present tense, and represents a particular goal or desire, such as *"Sitting the trot is effortless"* or *"My energy flows freely."* Sitting the trot may not seem effortless today, but using this affirmation will communicate your desires to your body-mind, and soon your positive statement will become truth. Utilizing an affirmation as a mantra is a powerful way to positively influence your state of mind, reduce fears and anxieties, and create desirable changes in both your yoga practice and your riding performance.

Mantras are versatile rider tools. Use multiple mantras during your ride to meet various needs. These can either be specific or general in nature. For example, you can repeat a single-word mantra such as *"Calm"* throughout your entire ride to overcome a sense of nervousness. While performing a specific riding exercise, choose a mantra that addresses your goal such as *"Hold the bend"* or *"Lengthen the stride."* Invoking one or more mantras, even if interspersed or used for brief durations, can greatly enhance your primary focus and help you achieve your riding goals.

Suggestions for single-word mantras:

• Breathe	• Balance	• Rhythm	• Fluidity	• Grace
• Focus	• Supple	• Release	• Peace	• Calm
• Relax	• Dance	• Give	• Allow	• Yield
• Harmony	• Oneness	• Union		

"The word mantra comes from man, which means 'to think,' and tra, which suggests 'instrumentality.' Therefore, mantra is an instrument of thought."[38] MARA CARRICO, *Yoga Journal's Yoga Basics*

"I always use mantras that are fun! 'Bouncy, bouncy, bouncy' is just fun! It relaxes me and reminds me to soften my joints and limbs as I repeat the mantra in rhythm with the horse's movement." VIRGINIA HILDRETH, *Yoga for Equestrians student*

Suggestions for mantra/affirmation phrases:

• I am light and supple as I ride.

• The horse and I move together in perfect harmony.

• I breathe in rhythm as I move.

• Riding is effortless.

• My body is both gentle and strong.

• I am calm and relaxed.

• I am a balanced rider.

• My horse and I dance gracefully together.

• Riding is yoga.

SECTION 2. The Listening Mind

"Control over consciousness is not simply a cognitive skill. At least as much as intelligence, it requires the commitment of emotions and will. It is not enough to know how to do it; one must do it, consistently, in the same way as athletes or musicians who must keep practicing what they know in theory."[39] MIHALY CSIKSZENTMIHALYI, Flow

Yoga for Equestrians emphasizes the importance of becoming a mindful and attentive rider by teaching you to observe and "listen" with your mind to enrich self-awareness and inner knowing. Your "listening mind" can enhance your performance as a rider and deepen your connection with the horse. With a listening mind, you become more receptive to feedback from the horse, your mirror. You can then purposefully cultivate positive, desirable qualities in the horse by establishing them first in yourself through yoga practice.

The Conscious Rider

An observant mind will also heighten your state of consciousness. By increasing attention to your thoughts and feelings on and off the horse, you can become more aware of how they influence your actions. With elevated consciousness, you act purposefully, rather than being controlled by habits or reflexes as you work toward fulfilling your goals on the journey to Union.

Are you a conscious rider?

A conscious rider...

• chooses to honor the horse by striving to become the best rider she or he can be;

• is dedicated to the process of becoming and embarks on a journey of self-discovery within the framework of becoming a better rider;

- "owns" both her shortcomings and strengths to better recognize the origins of her thoughts, actions, and non-actions;

- strives to become more attentive and observant—to listen with her mind—developing a deeper body-mind connection and heightened sense of awareness, clarity, inner balance, and relaxed calm, both on and off the horse;

- uses the powerful feedback from the mirroring process to cultivate desirable qualities such as balance, rhythm, and relaxation in the horse-rider team;

- is awake and open to progress, growth, and change, continuously evolving to embrace new techniques and ideas;

- is aspiring and determined, exhibiting the ability to persevere while working to accomplish both long-term and short-term goals;

- is dedicated and devoted to the disciplines of learning, riding, and life; and

- fully accepts responsibility for her progress and communicates with the horse in a spirit of compassion and partnership.

A Reflection

The horse senses and mirrors your every breath and movement, including the subtle changes in your body that result from your thoughts. No rider exists in isolation from the horse; even with a saddle in between, a sensory relationship is created as the rider merges with the horse—either in concert or in disarray. It is the rider's responsibility to infuse her alliance with the horse with qualities that nurture Union, not destroy it.

In the dynamic mirroring process, the horse receives and responds to the rider's stimuli. Nothing escapes the horse's sensory perceptions because a rider sits mere centimeters away from the nerves that pass through his spinal column. The quality of the rider's influence can fluctuate from harmony to disharmony in a heartbeat or a hoof beat. If the rider is tense, the horse becomes tense. If the rider is relaxed, the horse becomes relaxed. If the rider's movements are abrupt and unbalanced, how could the horse's movements flow? It is, indeed, a simple equation. Only when the rider has achieved sufficient levels of self-awareness, mental clarity, and physical balance, which enable the rider to communicate effectively, will the horse reflect the rider's proficiency and skill.

It is important to understand that the mirroring phenomenon does not distinguish between desirable qualities and undesirable qualities—the horse will reflect them all. Although the mirroring phenomenon reflects poetry when a horse is ridden by an accomplished rider, a novice may become disheartened by her horse's reflection, concluding that she does not possess the talent nor have the time and stamina necessary to bring out the best qualities in the horse. Take heart! The horse is a forgiving creature that graciously tolerates a rider's learning. See the undesirable attributes he may mirror back to you as lessons for you to learn. Allow yourself to mirror the horse's patient, charitable nature as you persevere toward achieving positive qualities in your riding performance through Yoga for Equestrians.

"Nothing exists in isolation. The old masters knew this well. This is the secret of yoga."[40] ERICH SCHIFFMANN, *Yoga: The Spirit and Practice of Moving Into Stillness*

"Through their uncanny ability to 'mirror,' horses spark a deeper understanding of our behavior, and inspire us to a more spiritual, mystical and philosophical orientation to life."[41] ADELE AND MARLENA MCCORMICK, Ph.D., *Horse Sense and the Human Heart*

Riding Without Force

"Blend compassion with authority...In your handling, seek a balance between firm and gentle."[42] CHARLENE STRICKLAND, *Western Riding*

The use of force in a riding lesson, whether by trainer or student, is counterproductive and inappropriate and does not encourage a competent, aware, healthy rider. Forceful riding may actually provoke accidents or mishaps that injure the rider and/or horse's body or psyche.

Whether under the guidance of a tactful instructor or on her own, the conscious rider eliminates the use of force in her riding by cultivating traits such as sensitivity, kindness, and compassion, which are inherently feminine in nature. Although these qualities have always been emphasized by the riding masters, they are often overlooked in everyday riding situations.

Polarities

As introduced in Chapter 2, yoga guides you to seek a balance between your Sun/masculine and Moon/feminine qualities. The conscious rider strives to cultivate equilibrium between these polarities in the saddle. Understanding the value of balancing these energies makes it possible to ride without force.

Masculine energy is active and operative, used to instigate change. It is with this energy that we physically *act*—on ourselves, as we urge our body past our edges in a yoga pose, and on the horse, through the driving and restraining aids. Masculine energy is also employed when you assert your leadership with the horse.

Sensitivity, cooperation, responsiveness, and receptivity are examples of feminine qualities. This energy is used to *synthesize*, or bring things together, as in creating a partnership with the horse. Feminine energy enables us to listen to our intuition and understand the silent communication of body language, both equine and human. This passive energy encourages you to let go of resistance and empowers you to *give* and *reward* the horse.

Yoga for Equestrians nurtures the receptive nature of the rider and encourages both men and women to weave more feminine energy into their riding. For most riders with traditional training, increasing feminine energy tempers the common excess of masculine energy that may result in aids that are too forceful. Using physical strength to make a request of the horse can tire you quickly and may irritate the horse or dull his response. Eventually, the horse may completely ignore your aids or develop dangerous vices such as rearing or bucking.

An overly feminine approach is just as unsuitable. Meek

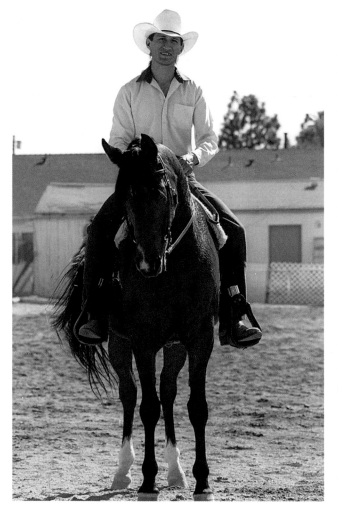

This state of quiet agreement is most desirable. It comes only when the horse and rider have mutual respect and trust and are in a state of harmony...such a state can never be forced. It must be earned and must evolve naturally."[43] DON BLAZER, *Natural Western Riding.*

attempts to direct the horse may seem ambiguous and vague to him. Too much feminine energy can result in lack of discipline or a disconnection between horse and rider. The absence of active leadership can give rise to a distracted, evasive horse. The key is to find the *balance* between masculine and feminine qualities, for herein lies the foundation of the essential "agreement" you make with the horse.

Ideally, this agreement is based on a balance of polarities, the circulation of masculine and feminine energies between rider and horse. You agree to provide the leadership, the guidance, and the intent, while the horse generously performs the work requested of him and, when treated with kindness, sensitivity, and respect, honors your leadership.

Yoga for Equestrians is an excellent way to foster balance between masculine and feminine energies. As you practice yoga, you are encouraged to treat your own body gently, without force, and to become more conscious, to *listen* with your mind as well as your heart while, at the same time, infusing your practice with perseverance, discipline, and strength. Taking this balance to the saddle will reward you with a partnership based on mutual trust that continues to evolve ever closer toward Union.

SECTION 3. Rhythmic Stillness

Rhythmic stillness is an integrated, harmonious state you can achieve during riding, yoga, or any rhythmical activity that engages you skillfully through discipline and training. When breath, mind, and body are focused, organized, and united in movement, you can experience rhythmic stillness throughout your ride, including the halt.

A Place of Peace

To achieve rhythmic stillness, you must first create a "place of peace" in your riding. Finding a place of peace involves overcoming stress to *consciously* develop relaxation in the saddle, which may require that you learn new techniques to shift gears and slow down. For instance, using a yoga warm-up before you ride can open the door to your place of peace. No matter what your riding level or activity, your place of peace is uniquely yours. It is possible to achieve it when you can accept where you are in the present moment without judgment. A place of peace can be found in the midst of competition as easily as on a trail ride.

Your breath is the avenue through which you can establish calm, confidence, and quiet control on the horse and discover your place of peace. As you consistently create inner peacefulness through yoga practice, you will bring peace to your work with the horse, who will reflect tranquillity back to you in his more willing, cooperative, and relaxed attitude.

The Use of Rhythm

While it is true that the horse moves with natural rhythm, if burdened by a stiff, unbalanced rider, the horse has a difficult time maintaining any rhythm whatsoever.

"You must be so in tune with yourself that you can function automatically, with your mind floating freely. You no longer have to try to achieve physical harmony with your horse, and, in fact, any effort to do so will interfere with the flow of your mind and block your spiritual unity."[44] JILL KEISER HASSLER, Beyond the Mirrors

We become a mantra that is understood by our horses."[45]
SHERRY ACKERMAN, *Dressage in the Fourth Dimension*

Understanding how the horse moves must be preceded by awareness of your own physical rhythms to enhance your sensitivity to the horse's movement and allow synchronicity as you ride. Ideally, the rider's body functions as a *metronome*✴ for the horse, keeping him consistent and steady through all gaits and transitions. This ability evolves when the rider fuels her own movements on the horse with her breath, integrating body, mind and horse in a rhythmical dance.

In fact, the only rhythmic system of the human body that is under both involuntary and voluntary control is breathing. This makes it an indispensable rider tool and, as your work with the asanas in the previous chapter has shown, you can consciously regulate your breathing patterns in concert with your movements. Mastering this in an unmounted setting will enable you to hold rhythm more naturally in your body on the horse.

Using a mantra silently or out loud while riding can also help you focus on rhythm to prevent your mind from wandering. Try humming or singing a mantra in time with the horse's gaits. When you ride, physical movements and breathing patterns can merge with the movements of the horse, so that *the organic, synchronous rhythm itself becomes your mantra*, absorbing your awareness and transforming your riding into a rhythmic stillness. As you strive to achieve conscious rhythmic stillness on the horse, remember this simple truth—by focusing on rhythm, you create rhythm.

Flow and The Altered State

"Flow helps to integrate the self because in that state of deep concentration consciousness is unusually well ordered. Thoughts, intentions, feelings, and all the senses are focused on the same goal. Experience is in harmony. And when the flow episode is over, one feels more 'together' than before, not only internally but also with respect to other people and to the world in general."[46] MIHALY CSIKSZENTMIHALYI, *Flow*

Yoga practice and riding are both activities in which disciplined involvement can result in an altered state of consciousness commonly referred to as a *flow experience*✴, characterized by feelings of being intensely focused or swept-up in the moment. Some feel enveloped in deep peacefulness as they skillfully perform an activity. Others feel elated—animated by the powerful, fluid currents of prana flowing through and around them, connecting them to their task, which they perform effortlessly and brilliantly. Many have described flow as a magical moment, a highlight, a peak experience, or a highly pleasurable moment of elation.

As you become proficient in your riding, the learning process shifts from the logical, analytical left-brain as the use of your creative, intuitive right-brain increases. This mental shift elevates the function and form of riding to artistic levels—inspired and beautiful. Although learning to ride requires that you process and absorb a significant amount of information using a logical, left-brain approach, once a skill becomes part of your repertoire, it is retained as a body memory, and becomes more automatic. At that point, you may experience a spontaneous flow experience. You might become aware of it only after you have finished your ride and shifted back into ordinary consciousness. In retrospect, you realize that you have participated in an extraordinary experience, an optimum level of performance in the saddle. It feels wonderful! And this sensation can consciously be cultivated.

Achieving a flow experience within yoga practice can enhance your ability to develop rhythmical stillness in the saddle. It is important to realize that achieving this necessitates more than mastering the mechanics of riding. Whether you ride for art, sport, or recreation, cultivating an altered state of consciousness is prompted by your strong desire for

Union with the horse. Using the techniques of Yoga for Equestrians, you may learn to consistently and regularly produce this flow as you progress toward your goal—Union.

Union

Attaining Union with the horse involves, for many, a spiritual union. In *Beyond the Mirrors*, Jill Keiser Hassler describes the experience of spiritual unity: *"Spiritual unity between rider and horse is...a union of their selves for the benefit of their performance together. The rider is no longer conscious of his own spirit, but only of the bond he has with his horse and of the movements they are performing together."* [48] A spiritual union involves losing a sense of Self. Many highly skilled riders may agree that their experience of Union occurs when they "surrender" themselves to the horse. It no longer feels as though they are two separate beings but rather one horse-rider unit.

To attain Union with the horse involves two bodies, two species moving together in balance, in concert, as One. Your horse-rider partnership encompasses spiritual unity as you ride unaware of your own body, your attention attuned to complete, fluid integration with the horse. During these special moments, time ceases to exist and your activities flow effortlessly.

Through disciplined concentration and effortless, efficient movement, you have achieved a rhythmic stillness in the saddle. While experiencing this altered state, your breath flows in rhythm with the horse's strides. Your body movements are rhythmical, effective, and organized. Your mind is quiet, focused, and alert. Adjustments to your balance and alignment are made intuitively. Communication with the horse seems almost telepathic, and your aids are invisibly subtle and deft. You receive the horse's movement with your own as though you were an extension of his body. A sense of inner peace and uninterrupted self-confidence envelopes you. Absent are fears, anxieties, and doubts. With mutual trust between you and your horse, you feel you can handle anything and accomplish everything. You enjoy the skillful, effortless sensations of your riding activities and the integration of your body, mind, and horse. This is the altered state. This is Union.

"...once we have tasted this joy, we will redouble our efforts to taste it again. This is the way the self grows." [47]
MIHALY CSIKSZENTMIHALYI, *Flow*

"There comes a day, and later on sometimes every day, when you feel that you lose sense of your skills. You become unaware of yourself, become oblivious to your aids and whatever your limbs, torso, and musculature are doing. You become absorbed in an effort that seems independent of your senses and so thoroughly effortless that it suggests a feeling of being in a dream where you can ride but for the first time without awareness of the effort. When you no longer feel what you are doing or that you are busy, you have entered the artistic experience." [49]
CHARLES DE KUNFFY, *Dressage Questions Answered*

PART III

Yoga for Equestrians

"Our asana, the classical seat, must find soft and supple expression."[50]
SHERRY L. ACKERMAN, *Dresssage in the Fourth Dimension*

CHAPTER SIX

Sphere of Influence: Power Center

CENTERING is a powerful technique that encourages wholeness and optimum balance on all levels: physical, emotional, mental, and spiritual. It can assist you in achieving mastery of both unmounted and mounted activities.

The path to centering on the horse is circular, involving you in your entirety. Yoga for Equestrians fosters your ability to become centered by developing self-awareness, relaxation, deep abdominal breathing, and the use of mental imagery. When you are truly centered, you are physically balanced and aligned, mentally focused, emotionally confident, spiritually at ease, and closer to Union with the horse.

Learning to center involves getting to know your *Sphere of Influence*✻: the entire central section of your body comprised of your pelvis, lower back, and abdomen. Awareness of this vital area—where the rider's upper and lower body merge—is important to developing your ability to center and establish balanced alignment on the horse.

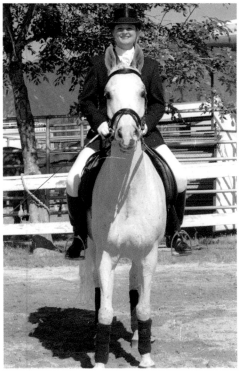

Centering is a circular process that involves you in your entirety.

SECTION 1. Your Power Center

The Sphere of Influence is home to your *Power Center*✻, the regulator of movement and energy throughout your body and the key to a great potential power within you. This power is expressed in enhanced self-control, balance, and poise when physical movements originate from your Power Center rather than your limbs. (Discussed further in Chapter 7, "Where Movement Begins.") Within your Power Center lies your *center of gravity*✻, located deep in your abdomen in your physical core: usually one to two inches below your navel and directly in front of the large, thick lumbar vertebrae. Later in this chapter, we will talk more about your center of gravity.

The Power Center serves as an internal *energy center*✻, conducting the flow of prana through your body (see Chapter 4) to animate and direct movement. In the yoga tradition, the lower abdominal area has long been recognized as the center where prana is stored and regulated. The Japanese define this area as the *hara*∗, *"the core or essence of your being through which you can experience an uninterrupted flow of coordinated energy, both physical and mental."*[51] This concept originated in China where according to Taoist principles, the practice of breathing centers the breath in the hara, which corresponds to the lower abdomen.[52]

Try the following visualization exercise to enhance awareness of your Power Center's energetic aspect.

UNMOUNTED VISUALIZATION: Power Center

1. Stand quietly and begin to breathe deeply. Close your eyes, flooding your Sphere of Influence— pelvis, lower back, and abdomen— with your breath. Focus your awareness on your Power Center, located deep in its core. Visualize it as the hub of a three-dimensional sphere swirling with energy, like a gyroscope. Picture the energy as vivid, radiating light and pause to experience it circulating within your Sphere of Influence.

2. Step your feet about shoulder width apart and slowly raise your arms straight out to your sides. Activate these spokes of energy with your breath and imagine the gyroscope enlarging your sphere of energy to radiate both within you and around your body.

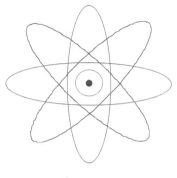

Gyroscope.

3. Continue to breathe deeply as you experience the prana that emanates from your Power Center pulsating through your body. Now, open your eyes and hold the sensation and image of your Power Center at the hub of this swirling, gyroscope of energy. Imagine your energy sphere expanding even further as your gyroscope becomes larger, swirling with the radiant, energetic light directed by your imagination. Feel how balanced and energized you are! Spend a few more moments visualizing this central area of power and the vibrant waves of energy emitting from deep within.

4. When you are finished, slowly lower your arms and return to a quiet standing position. Know that you can reconnect to your Power Center and experience this energy at any time.

Energizing your Power Center through the use of your breath will awaken and activate the prana within, enhancing your ability to remain centered, either on or off the horse. Centering serves as a foundation for fine-tuning and sophisticating your riding position and aids. As you master this ability, you gain a fundamental

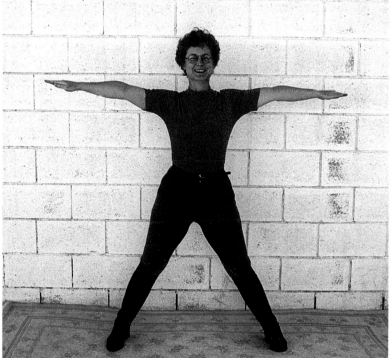

The energy moves within you and without you, and can be directed by you.

addition to your expanding repertoire of riding skills. The following exercise teaches you to "center" and prepares you for asana practice, promoting relaxation as it increases awareness of your Power Center's physical location. Centering Breath is a great way to take a brief time-out during a busy day, to regain a sense of calm in times of anxiety, and to prepare you for yoga or riding. With practice, you will begin to feel centered—not only physically, but mentally, emotionally, and spiritually as well.

UNMOUNTED AWARENESS EXERCISE:

Centering Breath

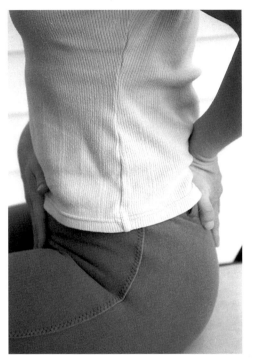

Centering Breath.

1. Sit comfortably on a chair, mounting block, or bale of hay. Place your dominant hand on the front of your body one to two inches below your navel. Place your other palm against your lower back, encircling your Power Center between both hands. Close your eyes and take several deep breaths.

2. Think of your hands as possessing a magnetic pull to draw your breath down into your Power Center. Breathe slowly and deeply, inhaling through your nose and exhaling through your mouth. Feel this entire area become energized as it expands and contracts with each Centering Breath. As you inhale, allow your abdomen to expand under your dominant hand. As you exhale, use that hand to assist the abdominals in pushing out all the air.

3. Continue breathing fully into your Power Center with an even, regular tempo as you reposition your hands lightly on your thighs. Maintain an awareness of the potent energy now circulating through your Power Center.

4. Allow yourself to enjoy the combination of feeling relaxed and energized. Stay here for as long as you like. To finish, slowly open your eyes and breathe normally.

VARIATION: Centering Breath can also be performed standing in Mountain (p.71) or sitting in the saddle (p. 162).

Center of Gravity

When you are breathing correctly, your center of gravity naturally resides within your Power Center. Incorrect or shallow breathing, which uses only the upper portion of your lungs, raises your center of gravity, often to your chest. A displaced center of gravity, or "top heaviness," increases the risk of mishaps in any riding activity. When your attention is focused on your Power Center you will be able to lower your center of gravity, increasing stability and balance.

Familiarity with your Power Center will enable you to correctly maintain your center of gravity during movement. Yoga for Equestrians teaches how to *initiate* movement from your Power Center to balance your body more efficiently and maintain your center of gravity deep in your core. When physical movements consciously originate from your Power Center, you will be able to move more efficiently and harmoniously both on and off the horse.

Riding From Your Power Center

While in motion on the horse, your center of gravity and your horse's center of gravity constantly shift. As you consciously attempt to remain in alignment with the horse through all gaits and transitions, the horse instinctively makes similar attempts to remain in alignment with you. Establishing and maintaining this harmony with your equine partner is a rider priority. If you are unable to remain centered on the horse, there is the distinct possibility that you will experience instability, loss of balance, and a sense of disconnection from the horse. In contrast, riding from your Power Center results in a more stable connection to the horse.

Keeping your center of gravity in alignment with the horse largely depends on his level of ability, as well as the degree of influence you have over the horse's body. Without sufficient schooling or gymnastic training, a horse may move awkwardly under saddle, throwing you off balance and making it more difficult to remain centered while riding. In the same manner, a rider can cause imbalances in a horse who may, in fact, be quite well-schooled but is unable to maintain his balance under an unsteady rider. It is best to learn how to ride from your Power Center on a horse that has had sufficient training and exhibits an adequate degree of equilibrium. As you become more skilled in riding from your Power Center, you will develop the ability to improve any horse's balance, stabilizing the horse's center of gravity to allow you both to maintain alignment.

As riding from your Power Center becomes more sustained, your ability to *regain* your center should it be lost during moments of upset will become very reliable. Drawing upon the centering abilities you cultivate in an unmounted setting will greatly assist during mishaps or spooks and help to lessen the likelihood of worst-case scenarios.

When you ride from your Power Center and bring the horse into balance, you are likely to experience an uninterrupted flow of energy circulating between you and the horse. As you include the horse in your energy sphere, be aware that the centered horse has a parallel ability to include you in his energy sphere. Your Power Center receives his energy, channels it, allows it to pass through your body, and recycles the energy back into the horse again. This powerful experience a rider shares with the horse can elicit feelings of lightness, buoyancy, suspension, and synchronicity. It is a true reflection of Union.

Cherry Hill, in her book *Becoming an Effective Rider,* suggests, *"...think of mastery as control with a subtle fluidity coming from your core and flowing in a circular pathway of energy around you and your horse."*[54] The following visualization expands upon the Power Center visualization (p. 67) and guides you in enlarging your gyroscope or energy sphere to include the horse you are riding. Once you are familiar with this unmounted visualization, try it in the saddle with an assistant holding your horse while your eyes are closed.

"This concept of the circular flow of energy can be applied beautifully to your riding; we can build energy deep within ourselves and then transmit it to the horse. The horse, too, builds energy and in turn transmits it to you."[53] SALLY SWIFT, *Centered Riding*

With practice, you can learn to use this exercise to reconnect to your horse at any time while you are riding.

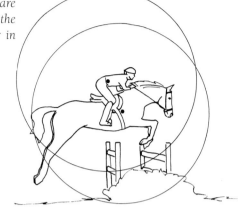

When you and the horse are centered, you each have the ability to include the other in your energy sphere.

UNMOUNTED VISUALIZATION:

Intertwine Your Energy with the Horse

In Easy Pose, close your eyes and become aware of your Power Center as you breathe deeply. Relax your mind and quiet your thoughts. Call up the gyroscope of swirling energy and radiant light from deep within the core of your Power Center.

Now, holding that image and sensation of your energy sphere, picture yourself astride your favorite horse. Imagine him in great detail as you perform your favorite riding activity together. Picture yourself in alignment over your horse's center, which lies behind his withers, deep in the core of his body. Visualize a similar swirling gyroscope of light and energy radiating from his center. Expand your energy sphere to include the horse's body as your two energy spheres become intertwined. Feel the mingling of energy; feel the connection. Affirm that everything within your energy sphere is balanced—your body, thoughts, actions, and horse.

Now, slowly open your eyes and maintain this sensation of your expanded energy sphere. Hold this awareness for a few deep breaths with your eyes opened and softly focused.

Using a Focal Point

"Let the object be the general center of your gaze, but look at it with your peripheral vision taking in the largest possible expanse, above and below as well as to the left and right. Be aware of the whole wide world.... Remember that you are still aiming at the central object."[55] SALLY SWIFT, *Centered Riding*

Your eyes play a very significant role in maintaining physical balance, allowing you to perceive the environment in which you are performing yoga and how your body relates to that environment. The asanas that follow can help you hone your ability to center and balance. Although many of the asanas and pranayama throughout this book may be performed with your eyes closed to help draw your attention inward, for the balancing asanas in this section we recommend that you practice with your eyes open.

As you prepare to bring your body into a pose, pick a focal point ahead of you, at eye level. Focus on this point with a steady gaze. At the same time, remain aware of your surroundings and the relationship of your body to your immediate environment. Expand your scope by incorporating your peripheral vision. You will find that your ability to maintain balance increases when using a focal point as you breathe into your Power Center and bring yourself gradually into the pose.

Practice keeping a fixed gaze on your focal point before, during, and even after you have completed each balancing asana. Experiment with glancing downward; you may find it more difficult to balance your body, or you may lose your balance altogether. Maintaining a focal point and a wide field of vision will greatly enhance your ability to perform balancing poses.

Your eyes are also used to maintain balance while riding. A focal point can assist in maintaining your balance on the horse while negotiating turns, diagonal lines, circles, and various patterns and straight lines in an arena. Sally Swift introduced the idea of riding with "soft eyes" in her book, *Centered Riding*. Swift recommends that you start by focusing intently on a focal point and then relax your eyes to look softly all around you. This technique is as instrumental in yoga as it is in riding and your practice on the ground will make it easier for you to accomplish it in the saddle.

MOUNTAIN

- Feet in solid contact with the floor
- Breathing is relaxed and full

RIDER BENEFITS:　Mountain is a fundamental position and the starting pose for most standing asanas. The rider achieves precise, vertical alignment of the entire body and a steadiness of form by centering in this simple standing posture. Mountain bestows a sense of power and strength as the rider establishes a stable, upright alignment. Becoming more familiar with the feeling of being centered will improve a rider's security and balance in the saddle. This pose teaches the rider to develop poise, centeredness, and perfect, effortless alignment.

1. Stand with your feet together, eyes opened or closed. Feel your feet in solid contact with the floor. Imagine them as roots growing down into the earth, supplying you with stability and nourishment. Maintain this connection with the earth throughout the pose.

2. Slowly bring awareness up through your legs, beginning with your feet. Draw in energy through the soles of your feet, into your calves, knees, and thighs. Allow your knees to soften; do not lock them. Draw energy up into your upright pelvis, aligning and balancing it squarely over your feet.

3. Continue drawing energy up through your spine. Balance each

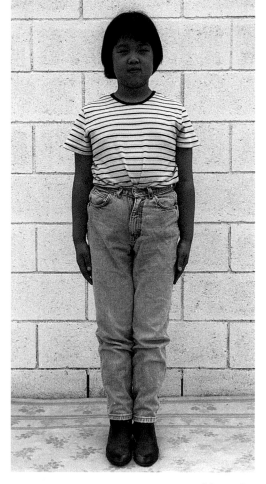

Mountain.

vertebra one on top of the other, all the way up to your shoulders. Roll your shoulders up and back, letting them come to rest naturally. Imagine a heavy velvet cape, or gentle hands resting on your shoulders, helping them relax down, away from your ears.

4. Move awareness up into your neck. Lengthen the back of your neck and bring it into alignment with the rest of your spine. Tip your head slightly forward and back, then side to side, until you find the perfect point of alignment that requires minimal muscular effort to balance your head atop your spine.

5. Breathe deeply and feel your feet in firm contact with the floor as your upper body lengthens freely from your Power Center. Notice how you feel. Enjoy this feeling of effortless stability and complete alignment through your entire body as you remain perfectly balanced. You are now ready to move on in your practice.

DANCER

- Lift through your hips
- Extend out through both arms
- Breathe into your center

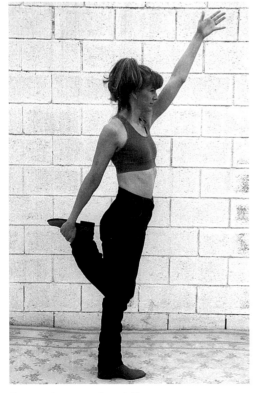

Dancer (see steps 2 and 3).

RIDER BENEFITS: This is a beautiful, classic balancing pose. Teaches the rider to develop the ability to remain centered through the slow, gentle movement of extending the limbs away from the body. Balance is attained through the rider's mindfulness of her Power Center, from where all movements initiate. Balance is sustained through achieving a dynamic stillness that cultivates strength and balance. Dancer sharpens a rider's mental focus through the use of the breath and visual attention. Physical benefits include a good stretch to the quadriceps, hips, abdominals, and chest, while strengthening the arms and legs and firming the buttocks.

TIP: Stand near a wall or fence so you can spot yourself if you lose balance.

1. Begin standing in Mountain. Breathe into your Power Center and gaze at a focal point in front of you at eye level to help maintain balance.

2. Shift your weight to your left foot. Bend your right knee and lift

your lower leg up behind you. Reach back with your right hand to take hold of the top of your raised foot. Keep your knees close together and your hips square. Balance on your left leg, focusing on your visual point to help steady you. Proceed slowly with awareness, initiating all movement from your Power Center.

3. Extend your left arm out in front of you and reach upward. Lift your torso up out of your center and elongate fully through the top of your head. Hold your gaze on your focal point as you continue breathing into your Power Center. Feel for your edges and remain here for a few breaths. Once you are balanced, proceed to the next step.

4. Press your right foot into your hand and gradually extend your foot upward as your torso pivots forward simultaneously from your left hip joint. Extend out through both arms as you hold the stretch, using your breath and focal point to maintain balance. If you feel comfortable, deepen the stretch as long as your balance is not compromised. Energize the lines of your body. Breathe deeply. Stay here for at least 2-4 breaths.

5. To finish, reverse the steps, maintaining awareness, until you are back in Mountain. Shake out your supporting leg and repeat the entire sequence on the opposite side.

Dancer (see step 4).

COUNTER-POSES: Standing Forward Fold, Straddle Forward Fold.

SYMMETRY

- Pelvis aligned

- Knees soft

- Shoulders relaxed down

- Smile!

RIDER BENEFITS: This asana, like Mountain, is simple, yet profound. Besides being a good overall strengthener for the whole body, Symmetry is truly an exercise in awareness. It will help you tune in to your Power Center and encourage you to energize your whole body with your breath. Symmetry teaches fundamental skills a rider will find invaluable in both yoga practice and riding.

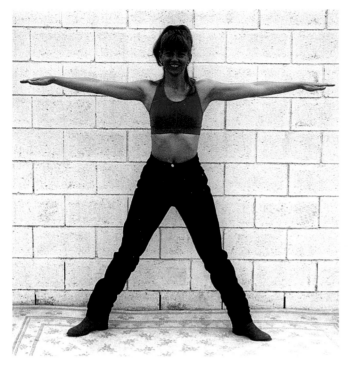

Symmetry.

TIP: You may find a full-length mirror helpful for visual feedback.

1. Begin centered in Mountain, then step your feet about 3 feet apart. Activate the lines of energy through your legs by directing prana down into the earth as you lift upward through your spine. Breathe deeply.

2. With a deep inhalation, sweep your arms out from your sides to shoulder height with palms facing down. As you breathe deeply into your abdomen, imagine yourself as a giant wheel with your Power Center as the hub; the lines of energy that flow through your arms, legs and spine as spokes on the wheel, radiating out from your Power Center. Fully energize your body with your breath, infusing each of the spokes on your wheel with vitality—all the way out to your fingertips and toes!

3. Be here for a minimum of 8 deep breaths. To finish, bring your arms back to your sides and step back into Mountain. Hold this feeling of dynamic centeredness and alignment as you move on in your practice or riding.

WORK IN THE POSE: Close your eyes and become aware of the symmetry of your body. Is your weight distributed evenly over both feet? Are your hips squared? Shoulders level? Arms parallel to the ground? Feel for these qualities first, and make any subtle adjustments. Then open your eyes and check yourself in a mirror. Are your adjustments sufficient, or do you have to align a bit more? Notice how your visual and physical feedback relate to each other—are they different or the same?

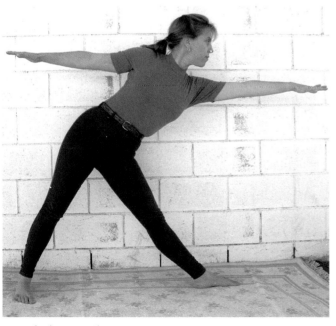

Triangle (see step 3).

TRIANGLE

- Keep the front of your body open
- Back of neck is long
- Legs energized

RIDER BENEFITS: Triangle energizes the entire body and increases awareness and control of the rider's Power Center as a source of prana to direct energy through the arms, legs, and spine. Triangle benefits the whole body,

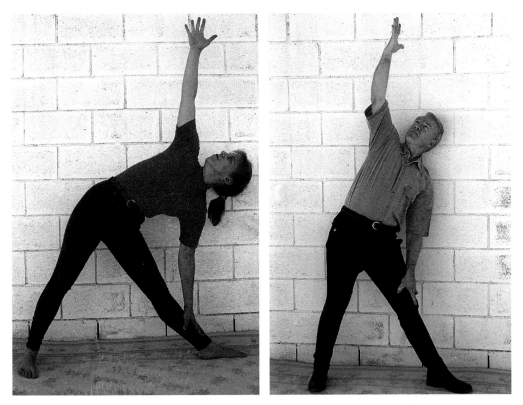

Triangle. *Triangle— Easy Variation.*

strengthening the legs and torso, opening the hips and chest. It gives a wonderful stretch to the muscles of the legs, torso, and arms.

1. Begin in Mountain, then step your feet about 3-4 feet apart. With a deep inhalation, sweep your arms straight out from your sides to shoulder level, palms down. Energize your legs, arms, and spine, just as you did in Symmetry.

2. Pivot your right foot 90 degrees to the right and your left foot slightly inward. Keep your torso and hips facing front. Feel as though your hips are opening outward. Feel both feet solidly in contact with the floor, pressing down through both heels. Throughout the pose, imagine that your body is between two panes of glass so that your head, shoulders, hips and feet remain aligned on the same plane.

3. Look out over your right fingertips as you reach through your arm and shift your torso out over your right leg. Extend through your spine and let your right hip drop down slightly.

4. Let your right hand float to rest as far down as possible on your right leg, maintaining the extension. Make sure to keep your hips and shoulders in alignment. If your torso has rotated forward, move your right hand higher on your leg until you can bring your hips back into alignment.

5. Extend your other arm straight up and look past your fingertips, keeping the back of your neck lengthened. Energize all the lines of your body—legs, arms, and spine— with your breath, flowing in all directions from your Power Center. Enjoy this

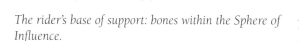

The rider's base of support: bones within the Sphere of Influence.

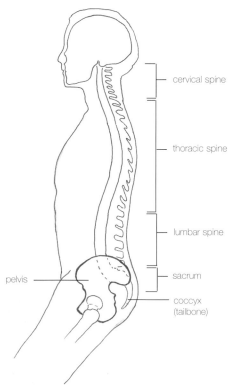

Ideal alignment: positioning your sacrum vertically ensures proper alignment of your pelvis, minimizing the curves of your spine and allowing vertical stretch throughout your upper body.

opening stretch throughout your body. Breathe powerfully and deeply here for at least 4 breaths.

6. To release, press down through your feet as you lift up through the top of your head and left arm on an inhalation, bringing your torso to center again. Release your arms, reverse the position of your feet and repeat to the left side. When you have finished, rest and center in Mountain for several breaths.

SECTION 2. Your Pelvis

Your pelvis, a supporting structure with your Sphere of Influence, is a large, dense, and very strong collection of bones resembling a basin. Many people have difficulty comprehending the true structure and position of their pelvis and are unaware of its influence on their balance, alignment, and movement.

Alignment, Awareness, and Adjustment

One of the main functions of the pelvis is to support the spinal column, making it fundamental to correct alignment of the spine. Discovering the sacrum, the lower portion of the spine which is jointed, or *articulates*✳ with the pelvis, is key to determining your own pelvic alignment. Becoming aware of your sacrum will familiarize you with your internal structure and help assess the alignment of your pelvis and spine. Bob Smith's *Yoga for a New Age* illustrates the relationship between the sacrum and the ability to correctly align your body. He states, "*the more vertical the position of the sacrum...the better one's chance of positioning the thoracic [mid-upper back] and cervical [neck] vertebrae in good alignment.*"[56]

Most riding students have been instructed countless times to "sit tall" in the saddle. The ability to comply is directly related to the spine's foundation: a properly positioned pelvis. If you have discovered that you typically sit with your pelvis either angled forward or backward, realize that you will undoubtedly sit this way in a saddle as well. Aligning and mastering the correct use of your pelvis while on the horse is vital to your development as a rider.

When the top of the pelvis is tipped forward it results in a hollow, "swayback" position that causes muscular tension and strain to the lumbar vertebrae. At the other extreme, a "collapsed" position results if the top of the pelvis tips backward, causing a rounded back and shoulders, collapsed chest, and protruding head and neck.

A tipped pelvis makes it difficult to find your seat bones and your vertical balance on the horse. Without a stable pelvis, attempts to correctly align your spine and "sit tall" will backfire, perhaps resulting in swayback or collapsed posture, rigidity, or top heaviness. The rider's position needs a secure foundation to effectively support the upright balanced alignment of the torso.

An upright pelvis is the foundation for the correct alignment of your spine, which allows you to receive the horse's movement. Correct pelvic alignment also increases awareness of your seat bones and enhances the development of an independent seat on the horse. When you have mastered the use of your pelvis and the muscular structure that surrounds it, you will be able to more subtly control your body and execute aids accurately and efficiently, improving your communication and performance with the horse.

Yoga for Equestrians encourages you to first firmly establish a stable pelvic position in an unmounted setting. Although sitting in a chair is certainly not the same as sitting on a horse, it is a good place to begin studying the alignment of your pelvis to become aware of how this influences your seat and your upper body in riding. As previously mentioned, ingrained personal habits can be challenging to change, making it difficult to establish the correct seat, even in a chair.

The following awareness exercise will acquaint you with your sacrum and guide you toward firmly establishing the correct vertical alignment of your pelvis and spine. You and your horse will benefit! Because you can actually feel your sacrum with your hand—the large, flat bone just below your lower spine at the back of your pelvis—you can easily determine whether it tips forward, backward, or is vertical. Use the illustration on the preceding page aand the photo below to locate your sacrum so that you can better understand and identify its alignment. It may help to perform this exercise in front of a mirror.

UNMOUNTED AWARENESS EXERCISE:
Find Your Sacrum

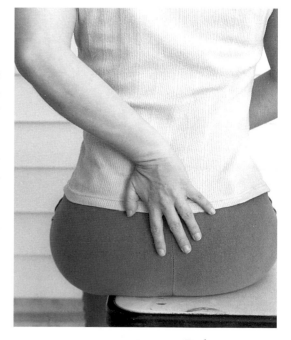

1. Sit comfortably on a chair, mounting block, or bale of hay. Place the palm of your dominant hand on the front of your body one to two inches below your navel. Place your other palm against your lower back, fingers pointed down. Breathe deeply and center.

2. Start to lower the hand that is on your back until you can feel the hard, flat bone of your sacrum beneath. (Turn your hand over if it is uncomfortable holding your palm against your back.) Notice the alignment of your sacrum. Do not make adjustments at this time; simply remain aware and open to the information your body is sending you. Continue to breathe fully.

REFLECTIONS: *Does your sacrum feel tipped forward or backward? Is it vertical? Can you visualize its relationship with your pelvis? Can you picture the pelvic bone within your body?*

Find your sacrum.

3. Move your awareness upward through your spine, vertebra by vertebra, through your neck to the base of your head. Become aware of any accentuated curves along your spine, especially in the lower back region. Take note of the balance and alignment of your sacrum, pelvis, and spine.

REFLECTIONS: *Notice how your back feels. Are there areas of pain, throbbing, or aching? Does your body seem heavy or light? Balanced or awkward? Aligned perfectly? Remember, yoga teaches you to accept where you are at all times.*

4. To establish a balanced sitting position, breathe into your Power Center, using your hands to guide your sacrum into vertical alignment. Direct your breath through your spine, extending upward. Release your hands and rely on the muscles of your Sphere of Influence to maintain this correct alignment of your sacrum, pelvis, and spine.

CAT STRETCH

- Lift out of your shoulders
- Reach up with your head and tailbone
- Lift through your middle back
- Release and open through the back of your neck

RIDER BENEFITS: Excellent for building awareness of pelvic alignment. Teaches breathing in rhythm with movement by coordinating the rhythmic motion of the pelvis with breath. Increases flexibility of the muscles surrounding the hips and supples the entire spine. When on all fours the rider can compare her body to the horse, and experience both a hollow back and a round back. Cat Stretch encourages empathy and compassion for the horse by increasing awareness of the strengths and limitations of the body.

Cat Stretch.

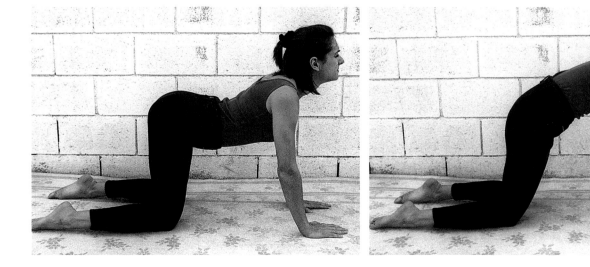

TIP: Use wrist variation (p. 31) if you have weak wrists, Carpal Tunnel Syndrome, or wrist injury.

1. Begin on all fours, your hands and knees aligned directly underneath your shoulders and hips—"a square halt." Notice if you place more weight on one hand or knee and then redistribute your weight evenly. Take a moment to think of the horse; relate how you feel on all fours to his ability to halt squarely.

2. Inhale deeply and raise your head and tailbone, letting your vertebrae dangle between them like a string of heavy beads. Lifting out of your shoulders, feel the stretch through the front of your torso. With your head held high, notice how hollowed your back has become and how this position is influenced by the extreme tilt of your pelvis. Pause here to observe how your body feels.

REFLECTIONS: *Imagine a horse with a hollowed back trying to carry the weight of a rider while in this vulnerable position. The further the back drops, compressing the vertebrae, the more the spine loses its shock absorbing qualities. When hollowed, your back is weakened and cannot effectively or safely carry a burden. Neither can a horse in this position.*

3. Exhale fully, lifting the middle of your back upward as you lower your head and tuck your pelvis under. Enjoy the stretch along your entire back and shoulders. Again, notice the tilt of your pelvis and how it influences the alignment of your spine.

REFLECTIONS: *When your back comes up, your head and "hindquarters" naturally lower. Your back is stronger in this position, with increased shock absorbing ability of the spine. It is easier to carry weight with a rounded back. Consider the implications from the horse's point of view.*

4. Continue for as many breaths as you like, letting each movement flow into the next. Follow the natural rhythm of your breath with your movement, inhaling into a hollowed back and exhaling into a rounded back. You can increase or decrease tempo while maintaining your rhythm. When you have finished, rest in Child's Pose for several breaths.

SWAYBACK

- Pelvis is upright
- Buttocks and upper thighs relaxed
- Extend upward from your center
- Abdominal muscles lift in and up

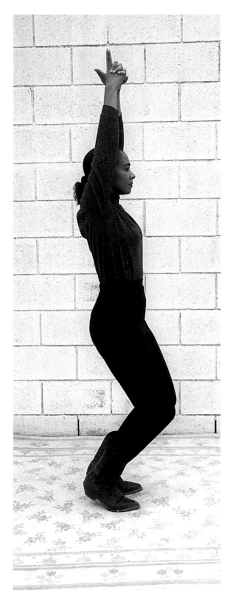

Swayback.

RIDER BENEFITS: Enhances the rider's awareness of pelvic tilt and how to adjust it. Strengthens the legs and improves concentration and balance. Tones the abdominal muscles, illuminating their role in pelvic alignment. Helps to correct or prevent a swayback position in the rider by addressing the relationship that often exists between weak abdominals and a tight lower back. Stretching the lower back muscles and engaging the abdominals enables the rider to reduce strain to the lower back and position her pelvis correctly both on and off the horse.

1. Begin standing in Mountain, correctly aligning your pelvis. Gaze softly at a focal point straight ahead of you.

2. Inhale deeply; sweep your arms out from your sides, then straight up above your head, interlacing your fingers with palms pressed together. At the same time, rise up onto your toes.

3. Begin to exhale; stay on your toes, keeping your arms above you. Slowly bend your knees and lower your body as though you were going to sit in a chair. Stay balanced in this position, tall through your upper body, and continue to breathe rhythmically.

4. Bring your attention to your pelvis. Continue to breathe and purposefully hollow your back, tilting the top of your pelvis forward into a swayback position. Now, draw your abdominal muscles inward and upward, bringing the top of your pelvis toward your spine without contracting your buttocks. Your shoulders, hips, and heels should be in alignment, as in Mountain. Be here for at least 4 breaths.

5. Come out of the pose on an exhalation. Straighten your legs and lower your heels. Let your arms float down to your sides.

6. Repeat Swayback several times. As you practice this asana, take time to experiment with the tilt of your pelvis to get a feel for the way your abdominal muscles affect its position.

COUNTER-POSES: Standing Forward Fold, Straddle Forward Fold

SECTION 3. Your Seat Bones

Although your seat bones are actually part of your pelvis, their role is so important to your riding we have dedicated this section completely to them. Whether or not you have been "formally introduced" to your seat bones, you can learn specific techniques to help you become familiar with them and better understand their use in riding.

Grounding

Grounding✳ is an exercise that involves both body and mind to connect you with whatever is below you: your seat bones anchor you to the chair, the saddle, the horse, the ground—whatever you are sitting upon—down to the very core of the earth. Grounding, a mental exercise that may begin with visualization, has a very tangible effect on your body. As you ground yourself, your seat bones may feel as though they have extended downward into what you are sitting on, as if "plugged-in" to the chair or the saddle. Your seat may feel "heavy" or weighted down as you use your imagination to create a *grounding cord*✳, visualized as a beam of light, a ribbon of color, a vine or root that extends from your Power Center through your lower spine and seat bones, into the earth.

Try the following visualization in an unmounted setting where you will be comfortable sitting for a few minutes. Chapter 10, Yoga in the Saddle, provides a mounted version of this visualization to assist you in applying these techniques while on the horse.

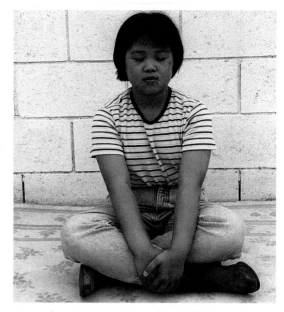

Grounding gives you the sensation of being connected and anchored to what is below you.

UNMOUNTED VISUALIZATION: Grounding

Begin sitting upright on a chair, mounting block, or bale of hay. You may need to sit on the edge to keep your body balanced over both seat bones. Breathe deeply and rhythmically into your Power Center and bring your pelvis and spine into balanced alignment. Plant your feet firmly on the floor and rest your palms on your thighs.

With your eyes closed, imagine or sense a cord of energy extending downward from your Power Center through your seat bones, your chair, the ground beneath you, and deep into the earth. Give this cord a form and make it real. Feel it connect you to the earth. The more clearly you experience your grounding cord through your senses— seeing it and feeling it—the more powerful this exercise will be for you. Perhaps you picture the roots of a strong tree reaching from your Power Center deep into the soil, nurturing you and replenishing your strength. Or your grounding cord may resemble a powerful gushing waterfall descending in a spray of blue and white. You might see a ribbon of swirling dynamic energy, depicted as color or light, linking your Power Center to the heart of Gaia, Mother Earth.

While holding the image or sensation of being deeply connected and anchored to what is below you, feel your lower body relaxing and melting downward, drawing you closer to the earth. Allow your seat bones to extend down into the surface you are sitting on, as though they were plugged in. Your lower body now feels comfortable and stable, no longer resisting the pull of gravity. Ensure that your torso continues to stretch upward from your Power Center. Your upper body should feel lighter now that you are anchored by your grounding cord. Being grounded has brought you closer to your root, to the earth. Your center of gravity and your balance are secure.

Bring your focus back to your Power Center with your breath. Slowly open your eyes, knowing that you have established a real connection to the earth and can reaffirm this connection at any time.

"...much of our physical and emotional discomfort is the direct result of a lack of connection to the earth."[57]
TODD WALTON, *Open Body*

Weight Shifting

"It cannot be over-emphasized that any shifting of one's weight must be so slight that, to the layman's eye, one is simply sitting. Too pronounced a movement is to be avoided at all costs. If one can be seen to have shifted one's weight, one has overdone it and the performance was bad."[58] WILHELM MÜSELER, *Riding Logic*

Learning to align, control, and distribute the weight of your body subtly and skillfully is a valuable rider aid. These skills both depend on and contribute to your balance and stability in the saddle, and promote a polished rider. Subtle use of *weight shifting*✳ and skilled control of your seat bones are characteristic of a highly developed seat. The rider who masters this aid exhibits grace, poise, and a refined position in the saddle.

At first, attempts to use weight shifting as an aid may feel uncoordinated; your movements may start out rather exaggerated. For instance, you may find that you lean excessively or collapse at the waist when weighting one seat bone. Do not lose heart! It is important to develop the ability to effectively shift your weight. This includes learning to center and align your pelvis, mastering the use of your lower body, and balancing your body weight squarely and evenly on both seat bones.

To use weight shifting effectively, a rider must have a sufficient degree of physical control and the ability to ride from the Power Center to ensure that the aids are imperceptible. There is nothing effective about overstated weight shifting aids.

The following exercises cultivate the ability to control and shift your body weight inconspicuously from one seat bone to the other without disrupting the integrity of your upper body, enhancing awareness of your seat bones in an unmounted setting to prepare you for yoga practice or riding.

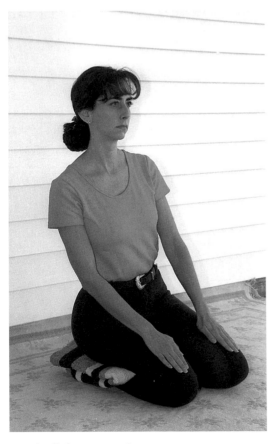

Weight Shifting – part I.

UNMOUNTED AWARENESS EXERCISE:
Weight Shifting I

1. On a mat, towel, or carpet, kneel down, then place a pillow, thick blanket, or a folded towel across your heels to provide a cushion. Lower your seat so that you are sitting on your heels. Your heels should be directly underneath your seat bones. From your Power Center stretch both upward and downward through your spine and allow your arms to relax, resting your palms flat on your thighs.

2. Breathe deeply into your Power Center and ensure your pelvis is balanced and aligned. Use your imagination to ground yourself. With each inhalation, reach up through your spine and upper body. As you exhale, stretch down through your lower spine and strengthen your grounding connection. Notice the pressure on your seat bones as the weight of your body rests upon your heels.

REFLECTIONS: *What you feel through your heels is similar to what the horse feels as you sit upon his back, with or without a saddle. (A saddle provides padding between your seat bones and the horse, acting as a cushion for both his back and your body without blocking the transmittal of sensation.)*

3. Begin to lean or tip your torso as little as possible toward the right without collapsing at your waist. Notice how little you had to move to feel your right seat bone pressing down heavier onto your right heel.

4. Return to your starting position and repeat this gentle weight displacement to the left. Stay grounded, extending upward through your spine so that you don't collapse at the waist. Keep your legs relaxed under you; don't tense them up to support your body. Center and ground yourself to maintain balance.

5. Return to center. Extend both of your legs out in front of you to rest.

The second part of this exercise is a little more challenging, requiring you to shift your weight subtly, using only your pelvis, without moving your torso.

UNMOUNTED AWARENESS EXERCISE:
Weight Shifting II

1. Begin as in Part I, sitting on your heels. Now, try to achieve a similar shift in your weight without leaning or tipping your torso. Stretch upward, and breathe into your Power Center. Isolate your pelvis as you allow your right hip to drop slightly, shifting weight onto the right seat bone and pressing into your right heel. Ground your right side more deeply and sink more weight onto your heel. You will notice that your left hip lifts upward slightly and lightens the left seat bone.

2. Return your pelvis to a neutral position, with your weight balanced evenly on both seat bones. Repeat this exercise to the left, shifting your weight by grounding more heavily on the left seat bone. Return to neutral.

3. Consciously and subtly shift your weight from one seat bone to the other. Keep your pelvis isolated; do not tip the torso or collapse your waist. Return to neutral and extend both of your legs out in front of you to rest.

REFLECTIONS: *You may find you have more control of one side. Remember it is better to make a suggestion to yourself to ground more deeply than to issue a command that results in your body working too hard. Too much effort can cause perceivable movement and/or muscular tension in the rider. The object is to conceal your weight shifting and keep it subtle. Yoga practice can help a rider overcome one-sidedness over time to develop balanced control of weight distribution.*

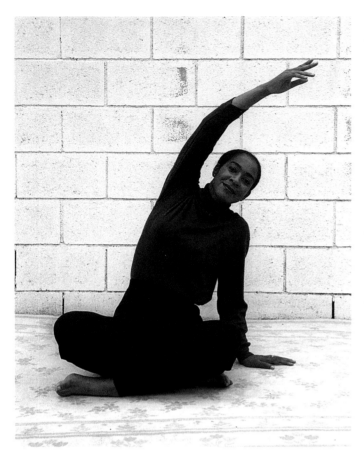

Seated Side Stretch.

SEATED SIDE STRETCH

- Keep an even contact with both seat bones
- Lift through your rib cage and sides
- Energize the arc created by your body

RIDER BENEFITS: Builds seat bone awareness. Encourages the rider to remain mindful of maintaining the appropriate weight distribution and connection through the seat bones. This awareness can carry over to mounted work, assisting the rider in remaining strongly grounded and centered while riding.

TIP: Use wrist variation (p. 31) if you have weak wrists, Carpal Tunnel Syndrome, or wrist injury.

1. Begin in Easy Pose. Center, breathe rhythmically, and ground yourself. Place your left hand out to your side on the floor or ground. This will be your supporting arm. Keep your elbow soft and slightly bent.

2. With one continuous movement, inhale deeply and sweep your right arm out to the side, over your head and to the left, creating an arc. Maintain your connection with both seat bones and the floor or ground. Let your head and neck follow the gentle curve of your torso. Extend and lift up through your rib cage to prevent collapsing at your waist. Feel a line of energy traveling along the right side of your body from your right seat bone up through your spine, through your extended arm and out your fingertips. Breathe fluidly and deeply.

3. Now, increase awareness of your seat bones. If your right seat bone has lifted from the floor, reconnect it to balance and anchor your weight equally on both seat bones. Feel a deep stretch along your entire right side.

4. Increase or decrease the arc by changing the degree of bend in your supporting arm. Keep your seat bones in equal contact with the surface you are sitting on as you adjust your upper body within the pose.

5. To release, maintain the extension through your right arm and spine as you bring your upper body back to center. Let both arms rest at your sides before repeating this stretch to the opposite side.

SPINAL FLEX I

- Reach forward with your chest
- Relax shoulders downward

RIDER BENEFITS: Spinal Flex improves rider awareness of the grounding connection through the seat bones during rhythmical movement of the torso. This is also an excellent asana for relieving back problems due to muscular tension.

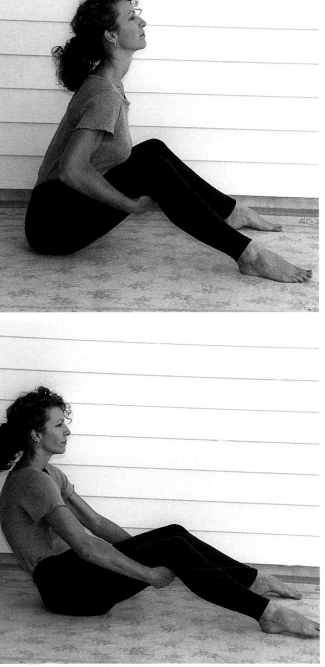

1. Begin sitting on the floor with your knees bent, feet flat in front of you about shoulder width apart or wider. Gently hold the back of your knees. Center and ground yourself. Choose a focal point to gaze at while performing this asana.

2. Tune in to your breath and begin to feel its natural rhythm. Feel it move through your body as you draw your breath down into your Power Center. Direct it down your spine and into your seat bones, then exhale completely.

3. As you inhale, rock forward onto the front of your seat bones. Gaze at the point in front of you and reach forward with your center and chest. Feel the stretch up your spine and out through the top of your head.

4. As you exhale, rock onto the back edges of your seat bones. Round your back and shoulders, and widen the space between your shoulder blades. Fully extend your arms as you pull back against your knees, completely stretching the muscles through your back. Keep your eyes focused on your visual point.

5. Continue this movement as long as you like, inhaling and reaching forward, exhaling as you pull back, rocking forward and backward on your seat bones in rhythm with your breath. Remember to keep your grounding connection in place. Rest and center when you are done.

Spinal Flex I.

SECTION 4. Your Abdominals

The musculature that comprises your Sphere of Influence—in particular, the abdominal group—is enormously important for progressing as a rider. This section focuses on the abdominal muscles, the "missing link" in the rider's ability to sit tall and establish a correct and effective position in the saddle.

The Role of the Rider's Abdominals

"...the use of the rider's abdominal muscles is rarely acknowledged, and...we hear far more about the workings of the back."[59] MARY WANLESS, *Ride With Your Mind*

The abdominal muscles can greatly enhance a rider's stability and security in the saddle by sustaining an upright pelvis. Sufficiently strong abdominals allow the lower back muscles to lengthen so the rider can maintain a balanced and relaxed position through all gaits and transitions. The abdominals perform several crucial functions in riding: they enable the rider to subtly execute transitions; aid in balancing and collecting the horse; assist in creating impulsion; help lengthen and shorten the horse's stride; and reduce and prevent strain to the rider's lower back. Abdominal muscles regulate the deep, rhythmical breathing that is instrumental for centering and grounding. They establish relaxation and the calm consistent rhythm in the rider's body necessary to develop rhythm in the horse under saddle. With such significant contributions to riding, it is a mystery why the abdominals have been largely overlooked.

Abdominal muscles that are weak and used ineffectively can't properly align the pelvis or protect the lower back from excessive wear and tear. Therefore, it is important for the rider to strengthen and tone the abdominals to bring balance to the opposing muscles of the back. In order to promote the rider's ability to initiate movement from the Power Center, the muscles that comprise the Sphere of Influence must be brought into balance. Mary Wanless advocates the importance of developing equilibrium between the body's opposing muscle groups and stresses that the key is to *"...increase the tone in the rider's weaker muscles, knowing that as this happens the tighter ones will let go, bringing the whole body into balance."*[60]

While this guideline pertains to opposing muscle groups throughout the body, it is especially pertinent to the relationship between the abdominals and the back. Increasing the strength of abdominal muscles is key to establishing a balanced tone in the musculature surrounding your Sphere of Influence. A strong set of abdominals may very well become the hardest working riding muscles in your body. Serving to keep your pelvis upright, support your back, maintain your center and grounding, deepen your breath, and help regulate your body's rhythm in the saddle, strong abdominals reduce the burden on the rest of your body and increase your ability to ride receptively and efficiently.

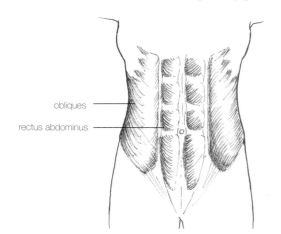

Abdominal muscles: rectus abdominus and obliques.

obliques

rectus abdominus

The Abdominal Muscles Defined

The abdominal group of muscles is comprised of the rectus abdominus, the obliques, the iliopsoas, and the diaphragm. (The illustrations on pages 86 and 89 illustrate their location in your body.) Because the abdominals contribute so greatly to your development as a rider, we encourage you to read the following descriptions to increase familiarity with this vital area of your body. Understanding and controlling your abdominal muscles is paramount to riding and significant to achieving virtually every equestrian goal.

RECTUS ABDOMINUS

The rectus abdominus runs vertically up the front of your body from its base at the pubic bone to its attachment at the front of your rib cage. This muscle forms part of the perimeter of your Sphere of Influence. Because the rectus abdominus is easily located, it is a good muscle to start with in building awareness of your abdominals. Place both of your hands on the front of your torso and notice how your rectus abdominus is influenced by your breath. When you breathe deeply and abdominally, it rises and balloons outward. After exhalation, this muscle returns to its normal resting place. Yoga practice strengthens and tones this muscle.

Weak abdominals are a primary cause for swayback posture both on and off the horse. Toning and strengthening the rectus abdominus, in combination with lengthening and stretching the lower back, is the best remedy. To achieve correct pelvic alignment, the rectus abdominus works in unison with the muscles along your back called the erector spinae. When the rectus abdominus contracts, the muscle shortens from top to bottom and the erector spinae lengthen, resulting in upright pelvic alignment. To correct and then prevent swayback, the rectus abdominus helps bring the seat bones forward and draw the top of the pelvis back toward your spine.

THE HALF-HALT

The synergetic action of the rider's rectus abdominus and lower back is vital to correct execution of both upward and downward transitions on the horse, as well as the half-halt, the important, momentary aid that precedes a transition. In *Becoming an Effective Rider*, Cherry Hill offers a universal explanation of this aid, *"In Western riding, the preparatory aid is called picking the horse up or checking the horse. This is similar to the half-halt in dressage: a calling to attention, a request that the horse reorganize and rebalance his body so that the coming transition will occur correctly and smoothly."*[62] Although the half-halt is a debated subject throughout the horse world, it is interesting to examine the Western rider's basic concept of a well executed half-halt, the aid that can create desirable changes in the horse's carriage and balance.

"Picking the horse up" begins deep within your Sphere of Influence with the cooperative action of the rectus abdominus and lower back. By engaging your breath to assist in executing a half-halt to check, collect, or rebalance the horse, the horse's back can be drawn upward with the lifting action of your rectus abdominus. As this muscle is contracted inward and upward toward your spine as you exhale, it helps to create more suspension in the horse's gait by inviting his back up. When the horse is centered, he naturally responds to this aid by elevating his back, seeking to remain connected with your seat. Influenced by the half-halt, he is now more attentive and prepared for your next request.

"As the rectus abdominus muscle is drawn in and up, the lower back muscles and the lumbar vertebrae quite naturally will lengthen. The pelvis is drawn under by means of a pulley system: the rectus abdominus muscles pull one way the erector spinae muscles go down the other way."[61] BOB SMITH, *Yoga for a New Age*

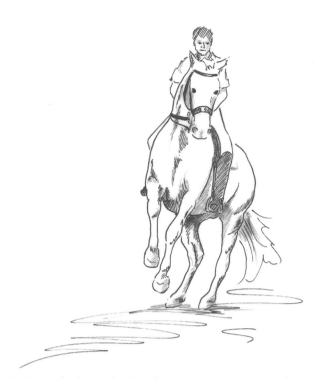

Raise the horse's back with more ease through the lifting action of the rectus abdominus, creating lightness and "picking the horse up."

With the rectus abdominus supporting an upright pelvis, you are freer to stretch upward through *both* the front and back of your torso once you are centered and grounded. The toned and activated rectus abdominus helps channel energy through the front of your body, contributing to the *lift* you need to sit tall or pick the horse up. When engaged rhythmically, this muscle coordinates with your breathing patterns and the horse's stride, assisting with the correct timing and execution of your aids. The specific use of a rider's rectus abdominus, whether occasional or sustained, will depend upon her riding style and goals. Riders of all styles who strengthen this very influential muscle will find it greatly improves their performance on the horse.

OBLIQUES

The obliques actually consist of several layers of muscles (see illustration on p. 86) located along both sides of your torso, near your waist, extending from your back to the front of your body where they meet the rectus abdominus. In concert with your back muscles, the obliques allow your torso to rotate, twist, and flex. Place your hands along both sides of your body to feel your obliques working in unison as you rotate left and right at the waist. The obliques are supportive muscles. When they lack tone, pelvic stability is reduced and posture diminished. Strong obliques assist in establishing and maintaining correct pelvic alignment and engage during exhalation. Strengthening the obliques can assist in developing deep, consistent abdominal breathing.

At first glance, the obliques may not appear important in riding, but their contribution to equitation is significant. Stretching these muscles allows you to lengthen through your sides to bring your torso into lateral balance. Together with the rectus abdominus, the obliques enable you to extend upward through your torso and sit tall on the horse. A lack of balance between the obliques of your left side and those of your right may result in the common tendency to collapse at the waist, which may go unnoticed until you sit on a horse! Sitting evenly in the saddle without collapsing is fundamental to an effective riding position and is greatly influenced by the strength and tone of your obliques.

If riding is the only physical activity you engage in on a regular basis, you may find that the hours spent sitting on a horse have not done very much to enhance your lateral flexibility; you may find it difficult to rotate your torso or flex your lower back to turn to one side or look back over your shoulder. In fact, without specific activities to improve your lateral flexibility, you may not be able to keep your body as strong, supple, and toned as it needs to be for the demands of riding.

Without the ability to flex laterally as you ride and to *sustain* that flexion throughout a lateral movement, the horse will find it difficult, if not impossible, to perform for you laterally. Thus, oblique muscles play an important role in developing a rider's lateral balance, a *prerequisite* for the rider to be able to develop the same in the horse.

ILIOPSOAS

This important group of abdominal muscles, integral in your ability to sit deeply on the horse, is located within your Sphere of Influence. You will be unable to touch these muscles because they lie deep within your body. Note that the iliopsoas muscles attach to the lumbar spine near the root of the diaphragm muscle, then extend down through your pelvis and connect to the top of your femurs, the inner thigh bones.

Iliopsoas muscles work directly with the other abdominal muscles as well as the lower back muscles, which are all involved in postural alignment and stabilizing the pelvis. Often, the iliopsoas muscles, overcompensating for weak abdominals and/or lower back muscles, become overworked as they attempt to hold the body in an upright position. When the iliopsoas muscles are overworked, they become shortened by excessive contractions and act to draw the lower spine and pelvis forward, contributing to swayback. The release of the iliopsoas muscles is a vital step toward correcting this postural fault. Bob Smith explains that, *"Only if the iliopsoas muscles relax and lengthen sufficiently can the rectus abdominus and erector spinae muscles work as they should to draw the pelvis under."*[63]

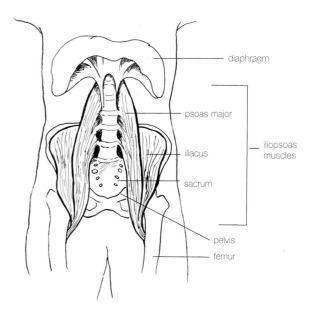

The psoas major and iliacus muscles make up the iliopsoas.

You can better understand how important the iliopsoas muscles are for riders by realizing that *the iliopsoas physically link your thigh to your lower back*, which is also an important conceptual connection in deepening the rider's seat. A truly *deep* seat extends *below* the rider's pelvis into the inner thighs, is wider than the seat bones, and is only possible when the rider releases the iliopsoas muscles along with the adjacent adductor muscles of the leg.

On the horse's back, the iliopsoas must be released to allow them to *lengthen* as your thigh is drawn down around the horse's body. For most people, this is a new activity for

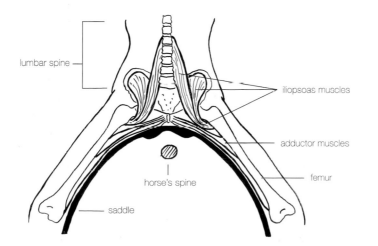

The deep seat: the iliopsoas muscles link your lower back and inner thigh, an important connection in deepening your seat.

the iliopsoas. Following their release, the iliopsoas must then be *strengthened*. In the saddle, they develop *isometrically* ✳ as they work to keep your body in place. When used properly, these key inner muscles enable you to draw the horse up under you and allow your deep, balanced seat to fully embrace the horse.

Practicing the abdominal exercises in this section will develop the appropriate balance, flexibility, tone, and fine-tune your control of the iliopsoas muscles.

DIAPHRAGM

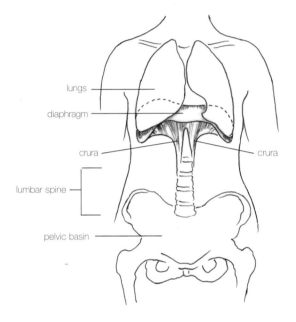

lungs

diaphragm

crura   crura

lumbar spine

pelvic basin

Your diaphragm is the muscle primarily responsible for the action of the breath. Becoming aware of your diaphragm is an important step toward making deep breathing an effective and instinctive riding skill. Located under the lower part of your rib cage, this large, central muscle is dome shaped, resembling a mushroom or umbrella. As you inhale, it draws downward, creating a vacuum, to fill your lungs. As you exhale, it moves upward, expelling the air out.

The "handle" of this umbrella is made up of tendons, called crura, which extend down and attach to the first four lumbar vertebrae of your spine. This is why, when breathing fully, movements of the breath can be felt all the way into the lower back and even around your sacrum and hips (see Breathe Into Your Back, p. 115). Your diaphragm rests under your lungs and heart, and affects virtually all your organs with each cycle of breath, bestowing far-reaching benefits. This is how your body was designed to breathe!

Deep, rhythmical, diaphragmatic breathing can assist you in remaining calm and centered on the horse through all gaits and transitions. Activating the diaphragm deepens your breath and assists in keeping your center of gravity within the Power Center. Bringing your attention and breath to your Power Center is an intrinsic function of your diaphragm, essential to grounding both in and out of the saddle.

ABDOMINAL LIFT

- Keep neck relaxed
- Lower back stays soft, receptive
- Relax your jaw

RIDER BENEFITS: Isolates, strengthens, and increases the elasticity of the diaphragm and surrounding abdominal muscles. Facilitates deep abdominal breathing and encourages it to become more automatic as the rider's muscles strengthen. Provides the rider a greater awareness of the internal breathing mechanism that is used in centering, grounding, and relaxation techniques. Increases tone in the abdominals to improve pelvic and spinal alignment and abdominal control to sophisticate and sharpen the rider's aids.

TIP: We recommend that you read through all the steps to fully comprehend this asana before you begin.

CAUTION: Do not practice this if you are menstruating, pregnant, have high blood pressure, a history of heart disease or stroke, or if you are wearing an IUD. You should practice this asana on an empty stomach.

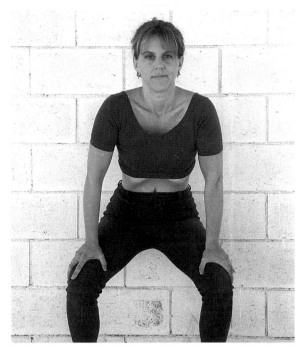

Abdominal Lift.

1. Begin standing with your feet about shoulder width apart or wider. Lean slightly forward from the hip. With your knees bent, rest your hands on your thighs just above your knees to support the weight your torso. Choose a focal point in front of you.

2. Inhale deeply, lengthening through your spine and out the top of your head, allowing your abdominal muscles to expand.

3. Exhale all the air from your lungs, then exhale even more as you draw your abdomen inward and upward toward your spine. Now, let your muscles relax to create a "hollow" under your rib cage. *Continue to hold the exhalation throughout the next step.*

4. Strongly push your abdomen outward with a quick thrust, then draw it inward quickly to create the hollow; without pausing, push it out again, draw it in, and so on, pumping your abdomen powerfully and rhythmically.

5. Repeat as many "pumps" as you can with your lungs empty, then inhale and rest in this position, breathing normally. Repeat the Abdominal Lift up to 4 times.

WORK IN THE POSE: Feel for your edges as you gradually increase the tempo and the number of "pumps" during each exhalation. You can gradually work up to more repetitions of the Abdominal Lift as you gain strength and control of your abdominal muscles.

BRIDGE

- Reach upward with your hips
- Open your chest
- Lower back presses into the floor

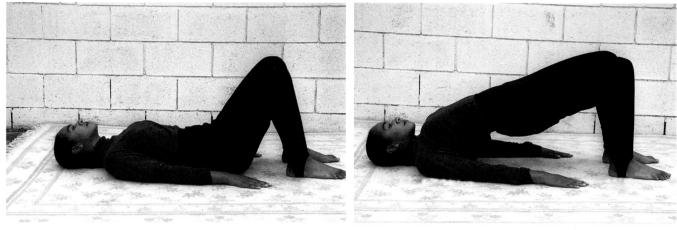

Bridge.

RIDER BENEFITS: Provides a good stretch to the entire front of the torso. Strengthens and tones the rider's lower back, buttocks, and thighs while opening the front of the body and stretching the abdominal muscles. It is particularly helpful for lengthening the iliopsoas muscles deep within the pelvis as well as promoting spinal flexibility. As a rhythmical pose, Bridge improves the coordination of the rider's breath and movement.

1. Begin on your back with your knees bent and feet aligned, hip width apart. Place your hands, palms down, by your sides. Feel your spine in solid contact with the ground. Take several deep breaths, allowing your breath to be rhythmical and fluid.

2. On an inhalation, in one fluid movement, tuck your pelvis and lift your spine, one vertebra at a time, off the floor. Leave your shoulders grounded and your pelvis tucked as you press your belly upward. Pause here and feel the stretch along the entire front of your body as the muscles in your legs, abdomen, buttocks, and back are activated.

3. Reverse this movement as you exhale, lowering your spine slowly down to the floor, one vertebra at a time, keeping your pelvis tucked and abdominals engaged. Relax your pelvis to its starting position, its full weight on the floor, then move fluidly back into Bridge on an inhalation.

4. Rhythmically flow from Bridge to your starting pose, completing a total of at least 4 cycles, moving in rhythm with your breath.

5. On your last cycle, hold your pelvis fully raised, stretching your hips as high as you can for a few breaths. Press down through your feet, keeping your knees in line with your hips.

6. Exhale, and descend slowly back to your starting position. Extend your legs out straight, relax and breathe normally.

WORK IN THE POSE: Your movements should be slow, fluid, and controlled. Let your breath guide you through this rhythmical pose.

COUNTER-POSE: Child's Pose

BOAT

- Extend through your spine
- Push out through the balls of your feet

RIDER BENEFITS: Activates and strengthens the musculature surrounding the rider's Power Center. Illuminates the inherent relationship between the rider's back and abdominal muscles: if one group of muscles is weak, the opposing group must work harder to sustain proper balance. It is common for the lower back to compensate for weak abdominal structure. This asana tones the rider's abdominals to bring these opposing muscle groups into balance, contributing to correct pelvic and spinal alignment.

1. Begin sitting on the floor with your knees bent and your feet flat in front of you. Grasp the back of your thighs, just under your knees. Breathe into your center and ground yourself. Extend upward through your spine.

2. Gently rock backward to balance on your seat bones, maintaining your center as you lift your feet off the ground. Balance here and breathe fluidly.

3. Maintain extension and stretch through your spine while you inhale deeply. Feel the muscles in your abdomen and lower back engage to help you maintain balance and extension through your upper body. Keep your shoulders relaxed and allow them to drop down away from your ears. Let your arms stay as relaxed as possible, keeping your hands in light contact with your thighs.

4. Raise your shins parallel to the floor. With your feet extended, toes pulled back, push out through the balls of your feet. Remember to keep breathing fluidly!

5. Release your hands and reach forward past your knees, your arms in line with your lower legs. Feel a current of energy emanating from your Power Center and extending out through your fingertips and the balls of your feet. Breathe and be centered here for 4 breaths. To increase the degree of abdominal toning, proceed to the next step.

Boat.

6. Gradually begin to open the angle between your torso and your legs by lowering them both toward the floor. Once you have achieved the position that is most appropriate for your level of ability, breathe deeply and be there for 4 breaths.

7. Rest and breathe in Easy Pose between each repetition of Boat, completing 4 or more sequences in all.

COUNTER-POSES: Cat Stretch, Happy Baby

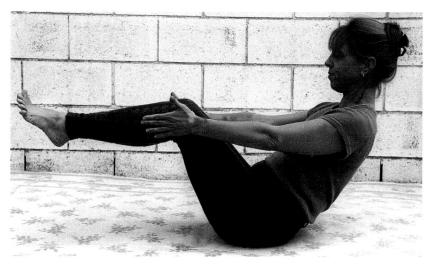

OBLIQUE STRENGTHENER

- Knees, ankles, and feet stay together
- Remember to breathe!
- Shoulders rest flat on floor

RIDER BENEFITS: This asana strengthens the oblique muscles and brings a healthy, lateral elasticity to the rider's body. Working the adjoining back and abdominal muscles to stabilize the torso is especially helpful in reducing a rider's tendency to collapse at the waist. Engaged obliques enable the rider to control and increase her lateral flexion, a prerequisite to establishing equilateral flexion in the horse.

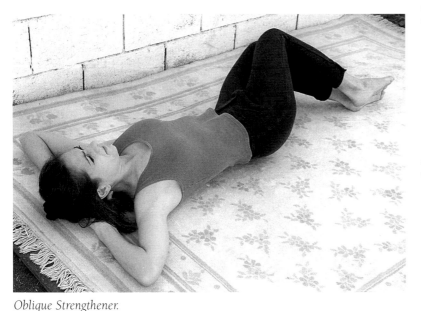

Oblique Strengthener.

1. Begin on your back with your knees bent and feet together flat on the floor; keep your knees, ankles, and feet together as one unit throughout the asana. Interlace your fingers at the base of your head, cupping your head in your hands. Breathe into your center and ground your spine to the floor.

2. As you exhale, slowly roll both knees as one unit toward the right, bringing them *no further* than a 45-degree angle to the floor. Keep the outside edge of your right foot on the floor but allow your left foot to lift slightly as you lower your knees. Do not force your knees down or allow them to drop toward the floor.

3. Look straight up, keeping your shoulders on the floor. Hold this position for 2 complete breaths. On an exhalation, bring your knees back to center.

4. Repeat to the left side. Complete 2-4 sets in all.

5. Hug your knees to your chest as a release. Take a few breaths in this resting position to finish.

COUNTER-POSE: Happy Baby

TOE TOUCH

- Press lower back into the floor
- Legs move in a smooth, controlled motion
- Keep abdominal muscles active

RIDER BENEFITS: This isotonic leg exercise relies on and develops abdominal strength, promoting higher muscle tone through the front of the body. Encourages fluid and deliberate control of the lower extremities and links this movement to the rhythmical regulation of the breath. Teaches the rider to initiate movement from her Power Center by bringing a heightened awareness to the abdominal structure.

CAUTION: If you have had a lower back injury, modify your practice of Toe Touch—touching only your toes to the floor without extending your legs—or you may wish not to perform this asana.

1. Begin on your back with your knees bent and feet flat on the floor, knees together. Place both of your hands, palms down, underneath your sacrum. Feel yourself grounded into the floor; allow your Power Center to anchor you. Take several deep breaths, allowing your breath to become fluid.

2. On an exhalation, draw your knees to your chest by engaging your abdominal muscles, pointing your toes.

3. On an inhalation, drop your bent knees away from your chest with a smooth, controlled motion and touch just the tips of your toes lightly to the floor. Immediately, start to draw your knees up toward your chest again, using your abdominals, as you exhale.

4. Repeat this cycle, each time touching your toes to the floor a few inches farther from your body than before. Use your abdominal muscles to move your legs as you draw your knees to your chest on each exhalation and extend your knees as you inhale.

Toe Touch.

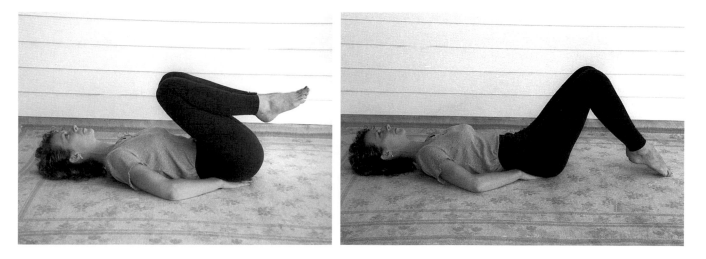

5. As you touch your toes farther away, you will feel the soles of your feet, and then your heels, come into contact with the floor as your legs reach full extension. Work slowly, with awareness, respecting your edges as you go.

6. Reverse the process once you have extended your legs as far as you can. Continue touching your feet to the floor with every breath, gradually progressing closer toward your hips until you are again touching the floor only with your toes.

7. Hug your knees to your chest as a release. Take a few breaths in this resting position to finish.

WORK IN THE POSE: The farther you are able to extend your legs, the more your abdominal muscles will engage, and the stronger they will become.

COUNTER-POSE: Happy Baby

❁

CHAPTER SEVEN

Connection and Symmetry: Lower Body

T HE RIDER'S LOWER BODY, in direct physical contact with the horse, is responsible for communicating the majority of the aids through the sense of touch. Most riders are acquainted with the active aids and use their seat, back, legs, and heels to influence the horse. But many riders need to develop the sensitive passive aids, which acknowledge the horse's correct responses to the active aids. Sometimes, the rider's most generous reply is to *do nothing*, rewarding the horse's action with a *non-action*.

Union is only possible when a rider's active requests are balanced with passive responses, such as receiving and yielding to the horse's movement. Unfortunately for the horse, these aids are often neglected or forgotten. A rider's incessant activity, whether conscious or unconscious, denies the horse space to perform or respond to her requests. For the horse to learn how to respond appropriately, the rider needs to be receptive and listen for the horse's response so that she can cultivate effective two-way communication.

Learning to yield in your yoga practice will promote your ability to perceive and acknowledge the subtle feedback provided by your own body, allowing you to become more sensitive to the horse's feedback as you ride. Forcing yourself in your yoga practice, as in riding, invites injury and pain and should be avoided. When you discourage yourself from overdoing in your practice, you learn to refrain from aggression toward the horse in your riding. Learning to balance these opposing elements, often at the same time, will teach you to approach riding more as a dance performed with an equine partner, moving you closer to Union.

In the previous chapter, we examined your Sphere of Influence, a very important area of your lower body, so

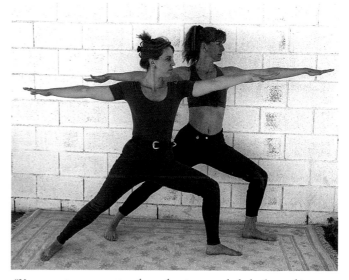

"Yoga creates symmetry throughout your whole body, making you strong and flexible in a balanced way. It also teaches you to balance the mental impulse to push, control, and be assertive with the complementary impulse to yield, surrender, and be passive." [64]
ERICH SCHIFFMAN, *Yoga: The Spirit and Practice of Moving Into Stillness*

fundamental that it required a chapter all its own. Now we will explore the rest of your lower body in detail, examining both structure and function in relation to rider goals dependent on the correct use of the lower body. These goals include deepening your seat, developing appropriate leg position and contact with the horse for balanced riding, increasing your ability to receive and allow the horse's movement, developing flexibility and symmetry, and enhancing your overall connection with the horse.

SECTION 1. Deepening the Seat

While most equestrians share the experience of sitting in a saddle, not all riders can boast of having a deep, balanced seat. Deepening the seat involves developing a closer relationship between the rider's body and the horse. A rider must learn to sit with feeling and sensitivity and to nurture the connection with the horse through all gaits and transitions. Even horses with a large repertoire of evasions won't dislodge a rider with a deep seat because she maintains a resilient connection with the horse's back. Acquiring a deep seat is the essence of a rider's journey toward Union and through the bond created by a deep seat, horse and rider appear as One.

Riders take note—no amount of money can buy you a deep seat. Expensive saddles will not guarantee it. There are no quick fixes that will enable you to deepen your seat in record time. No matter how badly you want it, you can't rush or force it. *Developing a deep seat will take time. Time and practice are essential components of your evolution as a rider.*

For the balanced rider of any discipline, deepening your seat depends upon your ability to open your legs out to the side and draw them back underneath you so that they fall directly below your torso and support the balanced alignment of your upper body over your feet. This is quite an involved process. Some riders may be prompted to try shortcuts, skipping through the basics. Keep in mind that even if you can recite underlying riding theory in great detail, intellectual knowledge is no substitute for doing the bodywork. In riding, as in your yoga practice, remember that the richness of experience lies in the process.

Acquiring a deep seat on the horse corresponds to your evolving ability to ride with *feel*. It is clear that the deeper your seat and the more you ride kinesthetically, the closer your connection becomes...and the more proficient you can be in any riding activity. Although this requires a great deal of actual riding experience, it is possible to prepare your body first through yoga practice to make the most of your time in the saddle. A deep, balanced seat is what connects your body to the horse and is a fundamental, yet complex, prerequisite for attaining Union.

Listen to Your Body

During the ongoing process of deepening the seat, pain in the muscles of the lower body may result. When a rider begins to work beyond her edges, intensifying her performance, she may experience what many refer to as "good" pain—when the muscles have worked a bit harder than usual but have not been injured. Tom Holmes in *The Total Rider* describes this as "...*the mild aching sensation you will experience during exercise as your muscles begin to tire. Many people learn to enjoy this tired sensation as it leaves a nice, warm feeling in your muscles, elevates your spirits, and is your body's way of communicating that you are working hard enough.*"[67]

The characteristic muscle soreness in the lower body that sometimes accompanies riding can be reduced and often prevented with yoga practice. Yoga for Equestrians helps to prevent injury and is an excellent remedy for many of the aches that an inactive lifestyle, infrequent or excessive riding can cause. As a rider warm-up, the gentle, slow stretching of yoga practice helps the tendons and ligaments of your body to release gradually, as well as the deep, interior muscles that play such an important role in maintaining a supple, close contact with the horse and a deep seat. A cool-down with yoga helps reduce muscle soreness resulting from a long or strenuous ride. Other activities like hiking, jogging, swimming, cycling, aerobics, or weight training may strengthen your lower body (i.e., buttocks, thighs, hamstrings, lower back), but generally will not encourage the elasticity, suppleness, and extensive range of motion required of a rider's legs, which must rotate from the hip joints in a unique manner to accommodate the width of the horse's barrel.

Although preventing pain and injury is always the best course, equestrian activities have inherent risks. Aside from the obviously preventable sources of discomfort, such as poorly fitting tack or clothing, pain experienced while riding should not be passed off as something that just "comes with the territory;" you should never be embarrassed to acknowledge it and discuss it with your trainer. If you are *instructed* to push through physical pain by your trainer, remember—it is your body that will be hurting afterward. Is complying worth a torn muscle or tendon? Pushing your body too far puts you and your horse at risk and may result in injury or a riding accident. Listen to your body to know when to ease up in your riding activities.

If you suffer from soreness, stiffness, or pain that prevents you from riding, practicing certain asanas may alleviate your discomfort. The therapeutic nature of yoga can provide relief from minor injuries involving muscular strain or exertion. Riders may be surprised to learn that gentle stretching can actually relieve muscle soreness in some instances—helping you to get back in the saddle more quickly. If you have specific concerns about pain, explore them carefully and obtain qualified health care assistance.

As you strive to deepen your seat, observe the information your body gives you with objectivity, releasing judgment about yourself and your riding performance. Listen to your body to determine what its feedback means, and respond appropriately. If pain intensifies while you ride, you may need to stop what you are doing, rest, or move on to something else. Don't ignore pain or choose to push through it; pay attention to your

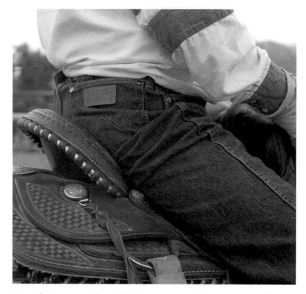

Developing a relaxed, deep seat is the essence of your journey toward Union.

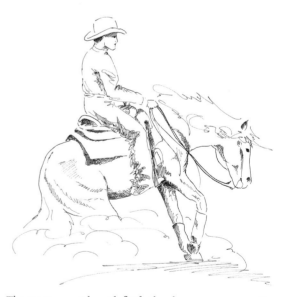

The more you ride with **feel***, the closer your connection becomes and the more proficient you can be in any riding activity.*

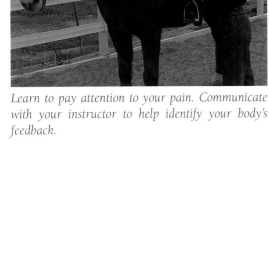

Learn to pay attention to your pain. Communicate with your instructor to help identify your body's feedback.

edges and listen to the valuable feedback from your body. Learn to be mindful of your body and pay attention to pain. Listen to your body, understand that your pain is a teacher, and identify why it hurts.

Meet New Muscles

Sitting on a horse may introduce muscles you never knew you had! The following key lower body muscles between your center and your knees are involved in deepening your seat. Familiarity with the muscles of your lower body and their function in deepening your seat in the saddle will help you to target specific areas of your body that would benefit from extra attention during your yoga practice.

ADDUCTORS

These are the inner thigh muscles that assist you in "hugging" the saddle and establishing effective leg contact with the horse (described in more detail on p. 108). Tight adductors prevent you from relaxing your legs and releasing your hip joints, resulting in excessive leg grip. In fact, if you squeeze unnecessarily with the adductors while riding, you reduce the range of motion in your hips (i.e. the "narrow fork") and thwart your own efforts toward achieving a deep contact with the horse. Compare this to the action of a clothespin: as the rider's legs close too tightly, they pinch her seat up and away from the horse's back. Clamped adductors also inhibit the horse's freedom of movement and restrict his shoulders, blocking energy and hindering his performance. A rider may occasionally need to employ the adductors during a ride over rough terrain, to help restrain a strong horse, or to prevent a fall or riding accident. Fine-tuning your ability to both engage and release the adductor muscles will increase the proficiency of your legs and help deepen your seat.

ABDUCTORS

These outer thigh muscles "widen" your legs and counteract the pinching, gripping action of your adductors against the saddle. The abductors (shown left) also assist in opening up your hip joints to develop effective, sensitive leg contact. The rider's goal should be to create sufficient muscle tone throughout the thighs as strength in these muscles enable you to draw your legs away from the horse's sides in varying degrees as required, yet rely on balance rather than grip to maintain a secure seat. Leg contact can be better managed and controlled through increased awareness of the abductors.

Yoga helps strengthen both inner and outer thigh muscles and

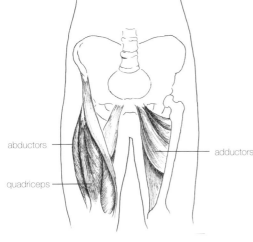

Leg muscles involved in deepening the seat.

complements traditional mounted exercises that involve opening your legs out to the sides and away from the horse's body. In fact, Müseler has recommended this type of on-the-ground approach for over 65 years! *"No amount of willpower, endeavors or strivings will prevent muscle stiffness returning if the legs are forced into the correct position. Exercises such as stretching each leg out sideways and straddling the legs wide apart can stretch the fork, or perhaps one should say the inner thigh muscles. But it must be emphasized that these exercises should be carried out several times each day...if they are to have any beneficial effect. There is no other way of improving the thigh position or of relaxing one's legs than by this kind of exercising off the horse."*[68]

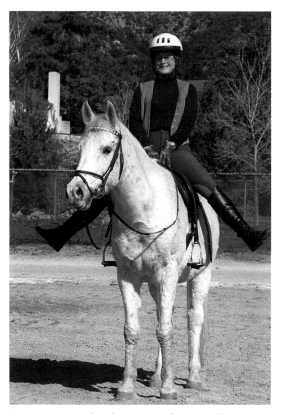

Yoga improves the elasticity and range of motion in the rider's lower body to accommodate the width of the horse.

QUADRICEPS

The function of the quadriceps (see drawing on p. 100) on the ground is to flex your thighs and draw them nearer to your torso, *closing* the angle at your hip joints. By comparison, riding is an activity that typically involves retraining these muscles, which are used on the horse in the opposite way, opening the hips. To maintain correct leg position in the saddle and deepen your seat, the quadriceps muscles along the front of your thighs must be both lengthened and strengthened to draw your thigh further away from your torso. Once the rider has released her hip joints and lengthened her thighs downward, the quadriceps must be strengthened isometrically to help keep both thighs in place. During this process, and often in response to a rider's instability or fear, the quadriceps may react naturally (but inappropriately) by drawing the thighs up higher on the horse in attempts to remain secure. This closes the hip angle, which usually results in lost stirrups and poor lower leg contact, as well as instability and imbalance. Stretching and strengthening the quadriceps through yoga enhances their integral role in riding and helps improve your position and increase security in the saddle.

HAMSTRINGS

The hamstrings are comprised of three distinct muscles located along the back of your legs. Important in developing your leg position on the horse, these muscles flex your lower leg (bend your knees), help lengthen your thighs, and open the angles at your hip joints. The hamstrings also assist in achieving the appropriate rotation of your leg for ideal contact around the horse's sides. Many riders have tight hamstring muscles and find it difficult to stretch them. In *The Runner's Yoga*, author Jean Couch offers a reason for this; the hamstrings

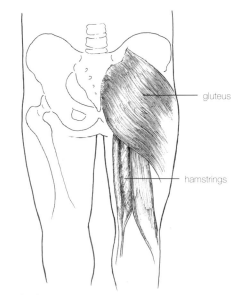

Lower body muscles involved in stabilizing the body and leg position.

"contain a high portion of tendinous fiber; one hamstring, the semitendinosus, is fully one-half tendon and tendons are far less resilient than muscles; like string, they are inherently resistant to stretching. This is why the hamstrings require consistent, patient work on the part of athletes and others who contract these muscles frequently."[69] Sufficiently stretching your hamstrings prior to mounting will enhance your leg position and contact and increase the mobility of your knees to prevent them from locking up while you ride.

GLUTEUS MAXIMUS/MINIMUS

The muscles of your buttocks (see drawing on p. 101) are involved in opening your hips, lengthening and controlling your thighs, and establishing the proper rotation of your legs on the horse. Toning the gluteus muscles will help stabilize your body in the saddle by providing you with a stronger, more stable seat. Deepening your seat involves developing greater awareness and control of your gluteus muscles to allow you to both soften your seat to the horse's back *and* act on the horse. Contracting or tightening these muscles delivers a strong driving aid to the horse, and it is important that you do so only with conscious control to avoid transmitting forceful messages to your horse unintentionally as you ride. Tense gluteus muscles can also stiffen your lower back, preventing a deep seat. Relaxed gluteus muscles can actually "spread" to cover more surface area of the saddle, thereby deepening your seat.

Release Your Hips

Yoga practice guides you in letting go of the tension and energy blocks in your hips that cause your seat to feel "locked-up." Your ability to consistently release the muscles surrounding the ball-and-socket joints where your thighs join your pelvis is important in deepening your seat and receiving the horse's movement through your lower body. Locked hip joints prevent both prana and movement from passing up your body through your seat and legs. Resistant hip joints create immediate rider problems and can lead to long-term rider habits that are difficult to correct. Yoga practice will teach you to release your hips and allow you to recognize the sensations of energy and movement traveling unrestrictedly throughout your lower body.

Your hip joints connect your torso and legs. When released, they allow your upper body to bend forward from this "hinge," balanced and supported by your stable lower body; picture a rider fluidly negotiating a jump. With released hips, your pelvis follows the motion of the horse's back and allows your legs to adjust individually to conform to the horse's body and maintain a steady, flexible position. Released hips enable your lower body to appear motionless in the saddle while in fact they move in supple harmony with the horse. Because of habitually contracted muscles, tendons, and ligaments around your hip joints, your initial efforts may result in only momentary release. However, with practice and experience, you can learn to reliably release your hips and stabilize your pelvis to receive the movement of the horse through all gaits and transitions.

As you practice the following asanas, become aware of the degree of flexibility in your hip joints. Use visualization and gravity to help relax the muscles of your seat. Scan your lower body to determine if your hip joints are locked up and resisting gravity.

Consciously release and relax the muscles surrounding your hip joints; create more space here by encouraging this area to open up through the use of your breath. With more freedom of movement in your hips, you may find you can eventually relax more muscles and deepen the stretch.

Remember to ground yourself before and during your practice. While you are grounded, release tension down through your seat bones and along your grounding cord in a seated pose, or through your legs and out your feet in a standing pose. While performing the asanas, imagine any anxieties, pressures, tightness, or discomfort that you may feel draining away through your grounding cord, into the earth.

COBBLER

- Knees reach down
- Release your hips
- Shoulders stay relaxed

RIDER BENEFITS: A gentle pose that brings an extensive stretch to the adductor muscles, opening and increasing range of movement in the rider's hip joints. Enhances the rider's ability to deepen the seat. Once comfortable in this asana, the rider can relax more deeply, maintaining it for longer periods of time to provide a greater release of the hips and increased inner thigh stretch. Cobbler helps to reduce stiffness and tension throughout the rider's hips and thighs.

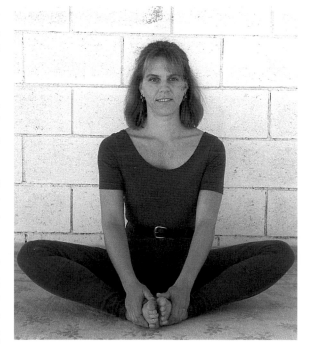

Cobbler.

TIP: If you have trouble keeping your back straight, or if you experience any discomfort in your shoulders or mid-upper back, sit on the edge of a pillow or rolled blanket to raise your seat bones (see Easy Pose Variation p. 35).

1. Begin in Easy Pose then bring the soles of your feet together, open your knees to the sides and cradle your feet in your hands. Draw your heels in toward your seat until you feel a good stretch through your inner thighs.

2. Inhale deeply into your Power Center to experience the fullness of your breath. Allow your chest to open and your shoulders to roll back and down. Extend upward through your spine, feeling lightness through your upper body.

3. As you exhale, draw your abdomen in and up toward your spine. Extend from your center downward into the earth. Let your seat sink deeply into the floor, grounding through your seat bones as you stretch your knees downward. Direct your breath to the muscles surrounding your hip joints, allowing

them to relax and open wider. Feel the increased stretch through your groin and inner thigh muscles. Relax your knees as you prepare to inhale.

4. Repeat this cycle at least 4 times, growing tall with each inhalation and grounding down with each exhalation.

5. To finish, return to Easy Pose and sit quietly for a few breaths.

HAPPY BABY

- Shins perpendicular to floor
- Relax and lengthen the back of your neck
- Ground through your sacrum

RIDER BENEFITS: This excellent hip-opener provides an intensive stretch and a deep release to the entire pelvic region and lower back. It increases range of motion and relieves stiffness in the hips. Happy Baby is especially effective in reversing the "clothespin effect" due to limited mobility in the rider's hips and excessive contractions of the adductor muscles. Assists the rider in establishing a stronger connection to the horse through widening the hips and deepening the seat, increasing the body's receptivity to the horse.

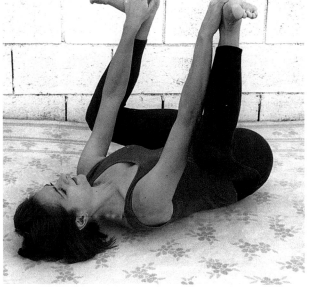

Happy Baby.

1. Begin lying on your back with your knees bent and your feet flat on the floor. Take a few breaths and feel your spine in contact with the floor. Exhale and bring your knees up toward your chest.

2. Extend your arms along the inside of your legs, taking hold of the arches of your feet with your hands. Open your knees and drop your thighs to the sides of your torso. Bring your shins perpendicular to the ground, the soles of your feet facing the sky.

3. As you exhale, feel your sacrum, shoulders, and knees drop down into the floor. Bring your attention to your hips; let them relax. Let go with each breath. Relax into this stretch and hold for at least 4 deep, relaxed breaths.

4. To finish, release your feet; slowly and gently bring your legs down to the floor.

WARRIOR I

- Shin perpendicular to floor
- Keep back thigh active, lifting up
- Chest opens upward

RIDER BENEFITS: This powerful pose is excellent for increasing the range of motion in the rider's hip joints necessary for deepening the seat and establishing correct leg position. Warrior I provides a generous stretch to the rider's hamstrings and quadriceps to help lengthen the legs down around the horse's body. Builds strength and stability in the rider's legs, gives a revitalizing stretch to the upper body, and helps to align the spine. Both Warrior I and II will develop the rider's physical balance, alignment, and control while enhancing the supportive qualities of the legs.

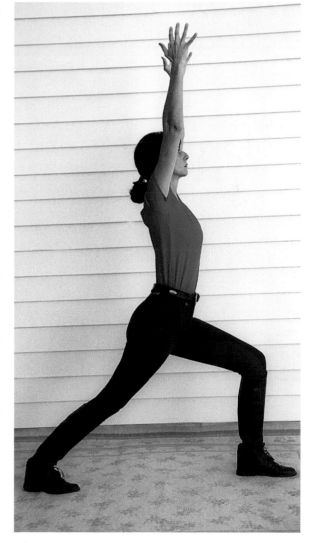

Warrior I.

1. Begin in Mountain. Step your feet about 4 feet apart, keeping your arms relaxed by your sides. Feel your spine lengthen upward as you ground down through your legs and feet into the surface below.

2. Rotate your whole body to the right, turning your right foot 90 degrees and your left foot inward about 45 degrees or more. If balancing is difficult, slightly widen your stance. Square your hips toward your right foot. Look down at your hip bones or feel them under your hands to help you find this straight alignment. Lift your abdominal muscles in and up, and let your tail bone drop down, feeling the increased stretch through your left hip and thigh.

3. As you inhale, sweep your arms straight up above your head, with your arms parallel and palms facing. Stretch your fingertips up to the sky. Feel your rib cage muscles expand and your upper body extend powerfully upward. Breathe deeply into your Power Center.

4. As you exhale, bend your right knee and let your hips slowly sink down until your right shin is perpendicular to the ground, stepping forward or back to adjust the length of your stance if you need to. Feel your hips drawn down toward the ground as you simultaneously extend upward from your Power Center. Keep your thighs active, legs energized, and both feet solidly grounded. Energize your whole body with your breath!

5. As you inhale, look up past your fingertips. Feel your entire upper body lengthen upward. Breathe powerfully and deeply here for 4 breaths or more.

6. Release the pose on an inhalation, straighten your leg, then exhale and let your arms come back down to your sides. Step back into Mountain, close your eyes, and take a couple of breaths to rest and center before repeating to the left.

WORK IN THE POSE: While in Warrior I, keep your neck and throat soft and relaxed, following the curve of your spine. Fill your entire body with your breath and feel your energy surging through you, grounding you to the earth. Feel energy flowing upward from your center through your spine, chest, arms, and out your fingertips, enlivening your entire upper body.

COUNTER-POSES: Straddle Forward Fold, Standing Forward Fold

WARRIOR II

- Shoulders relax down
- Front knee directly over foot
- Torso remains vertical

RIDER BENEFITS: As with Warrior I, this asana is ideal for increasing flexibility and mobility in the rider's hips. It is a particularly beneficial stretch for the inner thigh muscles, encouraging the rider's legs and hip joints to release and widen more easily in the saddle. Strengthens the abductors and gives a gratifying stretch to the upper body, helping to align the spine. Both Warrior I and II increase strength and stability in the legs as well as the abdominal muscles. The Warrior poses teach balance, alignment, and control—fundamental qualities in riding.

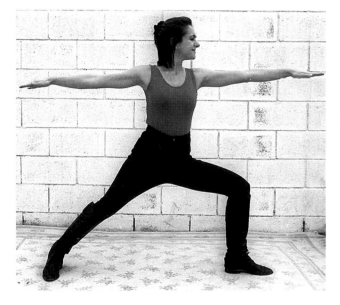

Warrior II.

1. Begin in Mountain. Step your feet about 4 feet apart, keeping your arms relaxed by your sides. Feel your spine lengthen upward as you ground down through your legs and feet. Feel the muscles between your ribs expand with your breath. Roll your shoulders back and down.

2. As you exhale, pivot your right foot 90 degrees and your left foot inward slightly, about 45 degrees. Align your pelvis vertically and do not allow your torso or hips to rotate; keep them facing forward. Feel as though your hip joints are opening outward. Keeping both feet solidly grounded, press down through both heels.

3. Inhale and raise you arms straight out to your sides at shoulder height, palms down. Stretch out through your fingertips, up through your spine, and out through the top of your head.

4. As you exhale, bend your right knee and adjust your stance until your right shin is perpendicular to the ground. Feel your right inner thigh muscle rotating outward so that your knee is aligned directly over your foot. Allow your hips to sink softly toward the ground as you extend upward from your Power Center. Ensure that your upper body is vertical. Keep your thighs active, legs energized, and both feet solidly grounded.

5. Inhale deeply, looking past the fingertips of your right hand, as your hips, shoulders, and arms remain aligned forward. Expand through your rib cage and feel your chest widen. Breathe deeply and powerfully into your Power Center, energizing all the lines of your body with your breath. Be here for 4 or more breaths.

6. Release the pose on an inhalation, straightening your leg. Exhale, letting your arms come back down to your sides, and step back into Mountain. Close your eyes and take a couple of breaths to rest and center yourself. Repeat to the left. Take a moment to enjoy the energy you have generated.

WORK IN THE POSE: Imagine your breath filling your entire body. Feel energy circulating throughout your body. Imagine the top of your head is drawn skyward. Relax as much as you can to ensure that you are using only the muscles necessary to maintain Warrior II.

COUNTER-POSES: Straddle Forward Fold, Standing Forward Fold

SECTION 2. Leg Contact and Postition

Your legs, when positioned correctly in contact with the horse, are the most influential tools you have to effectively communicate your aids. Developing correct leg position on the horse begins with learning to release your hips, as discussed in the previous section. The release process allows your thighs to lengthen, stretch, and drape down over the saddle to create large, open angles at your hip joints. Giving your legs to gravity promotes the deepening of your seat and your ability to sit in confidence and balance on the horse. Riding from your Power Center will anchor your seat, give you a greater sense of security, and eliminate the instinctive reflex to grip or hang on with your legs, which leads to positional problems and threatens your overall balance.

Once in the saddle, bend your knees to direct your lower legs back against the horse's barrel and align your heels directly beneath your hips. Place your feet lightly but securely in the stirrups, ankles flexed, with your toes lifted higher than your heels and lined up directly below your knees. Your entire leg, in contact with the horse's body, is now poised to communicate to the horse through the language of touch. To fulfill their role as *"the most important elements"* of your aiding system, your legs must develop the necessary qualities to establish and maintain the just-described ideal contact and position on the horse. These qualities include strengthening the appropriate muscles and ensuring that the joints of your legs remain flexible in the saddle.

"The rider's legs represent the most important elements of a harmoniously coordinated aiding system...They both propel (provide the necessary energy) and bend the horse. There are no legs without an anchored seat, and there are no legs without their independence of balancing functions. Legs should never grip the horse's sides in order to hang on."[70] CHARLES DE KUNFFY, Dressage Questions Answered

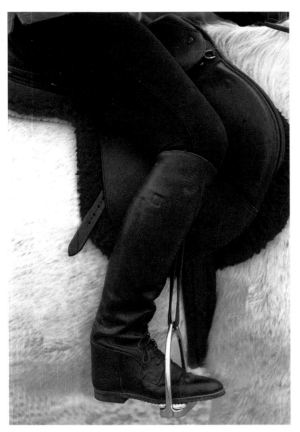

A toned, supple leg, in contact with the horse's body, is poised to communicate to the horse through the language of touch.

You may go through a great deal of trial and error before you establish the ideal riding position: ears, shoulders, hips, and heels in vertical alignment. This is the objective for English and Western equitation, as well as dressage riders. Be aware that if this alignment were forced, the result would be an artificial, rigid position on the horse that lacks feel. Rider's leg contact and position both must *evolve*. Yoga can assist you in developing a correct and effective riding position by improving the muscular strength and flexibility of your legs.

Hugging the Horse

The word "hug" describes the optimal way a rider uses the legs to touch and embrace the horse. Think of how wonderful it feels to be hugged, held warmly and safely in someone's arms. Now, contrast that to the feeling of being squeezed too hard, your rib cage squashed under a heavy embrace, enveloping you so that you can barely breathe! Imagine how the horse may feel between tight, constricting legs: trapped, pinched, and miserable. For the rider to hug the horse appropriately she must develop a breathable, *adhesive* quality in her legs, and master the independent use of each leg, as well as, establish independence between her upper legs (thighs and knees) and her lower legs (calves, ankles, feet).

Excessively strong upper leg contact can actually unbalance a rider, who may become top-heavy and lose her stirrups, tip forward or backward, or breathe shallowly or not at all, further compromising her position. Unless specific riding tasks require it (such as climbing steep hills or working over obstacles), chronically tightening the upper leg and pinching with the knees is counterproductive. Sadly, for both riders and horses, constant tightening of the upper leg is often *taught* to riders. This "short-cut" produces a false sense of security in the beginner and establishes an unfortunate habit that greatly limits both freedom of movement and stability in horse and rider, restricting the horse and sabotaging his performance.

When incorrectly or unconsciously tightened, the lower leg acts as an extreme driving aid. The horse may leap into a faster gait, his unaware passenger out of control. Gripping with the lower legs is a common mistake made by novice riders that, if not addressed immediately, can lead to accident or injury. More experienced riders who chronically apply lower legs heavily to the horse's sides can dull the horse's response and experience fatigue from the excessive physical exertion.

In contrast, floppy leg contact creates its own set of issues. Think of how irritating it is when someone bumps up against you repeatedly, or incessantly goes "tap, tap, tap" with their hand on your shoulder. A loose, swinging leg that repeatedly thumps against the horse's sides is not only very annoying, but in a very short time can cause the horse to ignore your aids and become "dead" to your legs altogether. Again, the horse can react by attempting to flee the irritation by increasing tempo or bolting. If your legs lack either the strength or flexibility required for the ideal adhesive quality, they will feel uncoordinated and swing uncontrollably from your hip joints, causing instability in the saddle.

Hugging the horse involves finding the balance between an excessively tight leg and an unruly loose leg. Because it is based on *feel*, it may take a significant amount of practice to develop. Through Yoga for Equestrians and specific mounted exercises, it is possible to gain awareness, balance, and physical mastery over your legs—skills that contribute to your ability to ride effectively, with feeling. Honing these skills will improve your ability to hug the horse with sensitive, communicative legs.

The equestrian must also develop an attitudinal balance between the use of the masculine *acting* qualities of the legs (the driving aids) and the feminine *receptive* qualities of the leg (the passive aids) to master effective leg contact and encourage the horse's optimum performance. Strong, sensitive thighs and calves can hug or close around the horse, or open and widen to yield to the horse's movements, as is appropriate during any riding activity. When your lower leg makes a request of the horse, an independent upper leg can soften, opening wider to free the horse's forehand as he responds to your request.

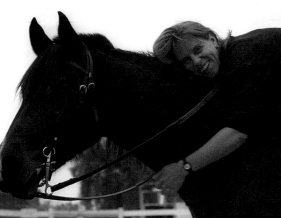

How wonderful it feels to be hugged!

Hugging the horse with a balanced, permeable contact—one that allows energy to pass through—enables your legs to develop the sensitivity to move in time with the rhythmical breathing of the horse. Yoga practice enhances awareness of your legs and conditions the muscles and joints necessary for hugging. With your legs softly molded around the horse's body, you and the horse can move as One.

Flexibility

Soft and flexible hips, knees, ankles, and toes, free from energy blocks and tension, allow energy to travel the full length of the rider's lower body. The ability to maintain correct leg position as you hug the horse depends on muscle balance, strength, and sustained relaxation through the joints of your lower body. Because releasing the hips is vital to deepening the seat, it was explored at length in Section 1 of this chapter. Even so, it is important to include the rider's hips along with the other joints of the lower body as we examine the desirable and necessary quality of *flexibility*.

Soft, supple, and elastic joints throughout your body allow you to *follow* the horse's movement. Your lower body must ideally remain stable, firmly connected to the horse by *isometric* contractions of your muscles while the joints function as hinges between body parts. The flexibility of your joints allows you to maintain purposeful leg contact and make the adjustments necessary to aid the horse effectively with your legs. Springy, bouncy leg joints play important roles in deepening your seat and establishing a secure and balanced position in the saddle.

If riding is your only exercise and you have been doing it for years, your lower body may be strong and firm, your joints elastic and springy in the saddle, but you may find that bending down to tie your paddock boots is next to impossible due to inflexibility in your legs or lower back. The tendons and ligaments that surround a joint are often difficult to release or stretch and, unfortunately for equestrians, riding doesn't do much to stretch them because the rider's position is relatively static. Fortunately, yoga practice *will*

"...experience shows that flexibility fades past the age of three in most children who do not bend and stretch regularly...Flexibility can be learned at any age through practice."[71] THIA LUGY, *Children's Book of Yoga*

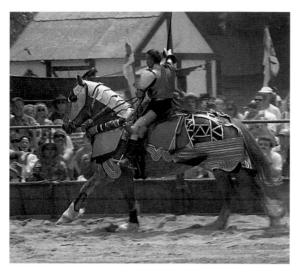

*Soft and flexible joints are what enable you to **follow** the horse's movement...even when jousting in body armor!*

stretch these important connective structures.

Riding does not involve much *isotonic*✱ use of the muscles; the rider's bones move very little during riding, apart from being lifted, dropped, shaken, or swung by the horse's movement. Flexible joints make it possible to absorb the horse's often unpredictable motion and channel energy throughout the rider's body to help her remain connected. Rather than clinging or bracing to remain in balance, the rider with soft joints can remain more centered as flexibility in her joints enables the rider to move in unison with the horse's back. Soft, elastic joints allow a rider to assimilate the horse's impulsion and suspension through the shock-absorbing qualities of resilient joints.

Yoga for Equestrians increases your ability to remain limber and keep your joints flexible. As you practice the asanas over time, the gentle stretching enables you to gradually remain in each pose a little longer as you progressively stretch out the ligaments and tendons surrounding your joints. Rhythmic yoga poses are especially helpful in teaching you to move with fluidity and grace. The holistic nature of yoga teaches that flexibility applies not only to your physical body, but to your thoughts and attitudes, as well. Being flexible means being open to change and new ideas, adding new methods and techniques like yoga to your riding.

Symmetry

Not many riders are ambidextrous. In fact, the majority are right-handed. This essentially translates into being "right-sided." You may not be aware of it, but as you walk, you may *lead* with your right leg, much like a horse's inside foreleg at the canter.

In working with the non-dominant side of the body, a rider may feel inept, lacking the finesse and fine-tuned control they have over the dominant side of the body. Many horses reflect this one-sidedness, mirroring their rider's strengths and weaknesses. Their stiff side corresponds to the rider's stiff side, their supple side to the rider's supple side.

Lack of symmetry is often apparent in the rider's legs. Ideally, both legs should hang down from the hip joints to hug the horse's sides, both feet balanced evenly in the stirrups. Eventually, the rider can develop the ability to use the muscles in each leg independently. However, for most riders, most of the time, one leg is freer to do this than the other. One hip joint tends to have more range of motion than the other. One seat bone bears more weight. One leg feels stronger, more able to influence the horse, and at the same time, is more resistant to "letting go" than the other. One ankle is more flexible, one foot more secure in the stirrup; the opposite ankle stiffens, regularly losing the stirrup. One knee grabs at the saddle more and is less able to release to allow the horse to move freely.

Lack of symmetry can exist throughout the rider's body, presenting a variety of challenges from head to toe. Addressing common rider challenges through yoga is an excellent way to achieve a more symmetrical body. Identifying the areas in your body that require more strength, stretch, or flexibility in order to match your right and left sides, will lead you to a better understanding of, and more empathy for, the difficulties the horse often has in complying with your requests for symmetrical movement.

PYRAMID

- Stretch out through your spine
- Front knee stays soft

RIDER BENEFITS: Provides a deep stretch to the rider's hamstrings, helping to supple the tendonous fibers that span the back of the legs. Assists the rider in opening up the chest while stretching the upper back and shoulders. Brings awareness to the alignment of the hips, teaching the rider to keep them squared. Increases flexibility in the hips, enabling the rider to lengthen the leg and achieve a balanced leg contact with the horse.

TIP: As you gain flexibility, try positioning your arms in Reverse Namaste (p. 141).

1. Begin in Mountain. Step back with your right foot about 2-3 feet.

2. Grasp your forearms or elbows behind your back. Make sure your hips are square, facing toward your left foot. Very slightly tuck your pelvis and feel the increased stretch through the quadriceps of your back leg. Breathe into your Power Center and reach upward through your torso.

3. Folding at your hips, bring your upper body forward with a flat back. Always keep the back of your neck aligned with your spine; move slowly with awareness. Feel the hamstrings of your front leg begin to stretch.

4. Continue stretching forward with a flat back until you reach your edge. Remain here for a few breaths. Feel the stretch increase through the hamstrings of your front leg as you breathe and lengthen through your spine and out the top of your head.

5. Now, fold down over your front leg and let your upper body relax; allow your back to release and your torso and arms to hang down loosely. Place your hands on the floor or on your front foot. This is an intense

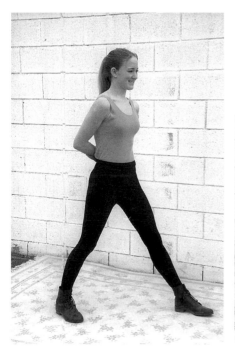
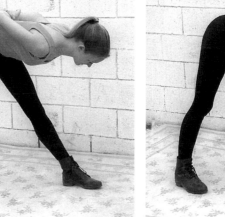
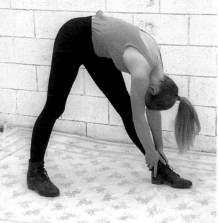
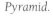

Pyramid.

stretch to the hamstrings, so really feel for your edge. Allow your front leg to slightly bend, then slowly straighten to help you ease into the stretch. Take at least 2-4 breaths here.

6. To finish, once again grasp your elbows or forearms behind your back. Straighten and lift your back, directing your breath through the length of your spine and out the top of your head as you come up slowly, back to an upright position.

7. Repeat on the opposite side. To finish, release your arms and center in Mountain for 2-3 breaths.

STRADDLE FORWARD FOLD AND ROTATION

- Lengthen through your spine
- Keep feet parallel

RIDER BENEFITS: Increases elasticity of the rider's leg joints, softening the hips, knees, and ankles. Provides a deep stretch for the hamstrings and adductor muscles. Helps lengthen the rider's spine and release the back muscles through the natural pull of gravity. The rotation relieves tension in the torso and opens the chest. Being a partially inverted posture, this forward fold is rejuvenating and increases blood flow to the brain, sharpening mental focus.

1. Begin in Mountain. Step your feet about 4 feet apart, your toes pointing straight ahead. Keep your knees soft, not locked. Inhale deeply and stretch up through your torso. Feel tall and light as you ground down through your legs and feet.

2. As you exhale, in one sweeping motion, fold at the hips, keeping your back flat as your torso reaches forward and down. Let your arms float down as your torso hangs freely. Place your palms on the ground if you can.

3. Let gravity take the weight of your upper body; breathe deeply and softly. Gently roll your head side-to-side to help your neck and upper back release. Allow the muscles throughout your back and hips to relax as much as possible. Let your breath help you release more with each exhalation.

4. Walk your hands toward one foot to create more stretch for the inner leg (if you can't reach your foot, place your hands on your lower leg). Feel the increased stretch through your inner thigh. If you don't feel any change, step farther apart until you feel your adductors stretch. Take 2 or more breaths. Walk your hands to the other side and take 2 or more breaths there, then come back to center. To move into Rotation, proceed to Step 6.

5. To finish, bend your knees and slowly roll up one vertebra at a time. This will protect your back and avoid dizziness as you return to an upright position.

ROTATION:

6. Place your left palm flat on the floor directly below your face. Straighten your left arm and extend out through the top of your head, creating a line of energy along the length of your spine, resulting in a flat back.

7. With a deep inhalation, sweep your right arm straight up to the sky. Keeping the back of your neck long, look up and reach through both arms. Feel your spine unwind into this wonderful rotation. Take 4 or more breaths here. Repeat to the other side.

8. To finish, lower your arm to the floor, then bend your knees and slowly roll up one vertebra at a time to protect your back from strain and prevent dizziness.

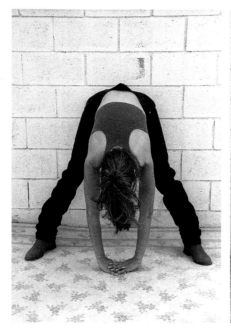
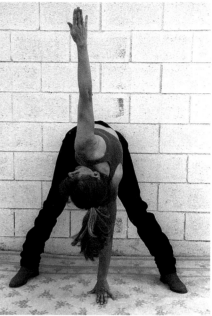

Straddle Forward Fold and Rotation.

TWO-POINT POSE

- Flat, extended back
- Neck and jaw stay relaxed
- Breathe into your Power Center

Two-Point Pose.

RIDER BENEFITS: Like the mounted version of this position, Two-Point Pose supples the rider's knees, hips, and ankle joints to help develop correct leg position. This deep stretch encourages flexibility in the joints to enhance the shock-absorbing qualities necessary to receive the horse's movement. Opens the hip joints. An outstanding strengthener for the thighs, calves, and ankles. Fine-tunes the rider's balance.

1. Begin in Mountain. Step your feet about shoulder width apart or wider, your toes

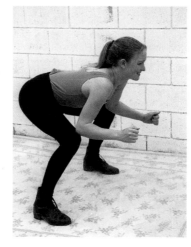
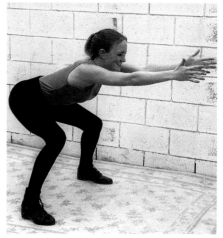

pointed straight ahead; knees soft, not locked.

2. Squat down and bring your elbows to rest on your knees. Close your hands in a soft fist as if you were holding the reins. Keep your back flat.

3. Inhale and extend your arms straight out in front of you, palms facing each other, your fingers spread and energized. Keep your back flat by drawing your abdominals in and up.

4. Continue to breathe powerfully in this position, activating the lines of energy through your legs and upper body as you stretch out through your spine and arms.

5. Rock very slightly forward and backward on your feet, feeling for the point at which you begin to lose your balance. Fine-tune your balance as you stabilize your position.

6. To finish, bring your elbows back to your knees, then slowly roll up one vertebra at a time. Straighten your legs and bring your arms back down to your sides in Mountain.

SECTION 3. Allowing and Receiving

Effective equitation is achieved by balancing active aids with a greater ability to receive the horse's movement and energy – creating a dynamic, yet subtle, kinesthetic communication with the horse. (Photo: Kristina Malmgren)

Many riders mistakenly *freeze* their body upright while attempting to influence the horse, often with mechanical and stilted results. *Effective* equitation is achieved by generating a *dynamic* position on the horse—one that allows the rider to both influence and receive the horse's movement. While a conscious rider balances the masculine forces that *act* on the horse with the feminine energies that *allow* the horse to respond, what keeps a rider consistently and correctly positioned in the saddle is the enhanced ability to allow and receive the horse's energy and movement.

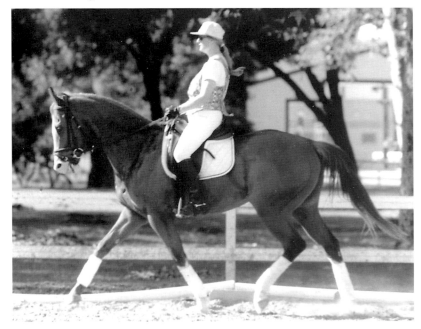

Receive the Horse

Every part of the rider's body can receive the horse in varying degrees. The seat and legs receive the horse's energy by minimizing physical activity. The hands receive the horse through elastic contact that channels energy forward through the arms, hands, and reins to the bit. The rider's lower back receives by yielding which, in turn, encourages the horse's back to relax, elevate, and soften to the rider. In fact, receiving is a vital function of the rider's back, requiring balanced muscle tone and flexibility.

A rigid, unyielding back may result from injury, inactivity, lack of confidence, fears, anxieties, or poor postural habits, creating significant energy blocks and causing the rider to brace against the horse's movements. The mild, rhythmical movement of riding at slow, easy paces may gently release these energy blocks. Yoga practice can also help increase or regain both flexibility and strength in your back.

For the rider to receive the energy and motion of the horse, it is imperative that flexibility of the back be developed and enhanced. A rider who can allow and receive the horse, encourages the horse to move more freely through his back. The asanas in this section will supple and strengthen your entire back, specifically targeting the important lower back area that not only receives the horse but is crucial in directly influencing the horse.

Through the Back

"Through the back" refers to the horse moving with forward energy that originates from the hindquarters and passes unrestrictedly through his back. Progressive training encourages the horse to use his back gymnastically while carrying a rider, an ability fundamental to dressage. A horse can only move through the back when the rider has acquired this skill in her own body. A rider can learn to move through the back once she understands how to *receive* the horse.

We go about our daily lives without much awareness of our spine or back muscles, unless, of course, they cause us pain or discomfort. To improve the quality of your movement both on and off the horse, it is vital to become more mindful of your back. Yoga for Equestrians is an excellent practice to develop the relaxation, suppleness, flexibility, and alignment that will promote your ability to ride through your back and consistently generate *throughness* on the horse. The horse will then reflect these same qualities back to you.

Try the following exercise to awaken a greater awareness of your back.

UNMOUNTED AWARENESS EXERCISE: Breathe into Your Back

1. Begin in Child's Pose (see p. 33-34). Relax and breathe deeply.

2. Tune in to your breath, feeling its natural rhythm. Notice how your body moves to accommodate the flow of your breath. Feel the rise and fall of your back as you inhale and exhale.

3. Focus your awareness on how your back moves in response to your breath. Notice the gentle, flowing movement of your spine. As you breathe, feel your lower, middle, and upper back expand with each inhalation.

4. Briefly place your palm on your sacrum and feel how this area widens when you breathe deeply into your Power Center. Now, feel your rib cage and mid-back expand. Notice how your upper back responds to your breath, how your shoulder blades move apart and up with each inhalation. Become increasingly aware of all the subtle movements occurring throughout your entire back.

5. As your back muscles soften, feel your spine softly yield, moving with your breath. Breathe more deeply to generate increased movement through your back. Feel waves of prana flowing through the curves of your spine with each breath. Be present with these sensations and enjoy this new awareness.

6. To finish, come upright very slowly, sitting on your heels. Be still for several breaths, breathing into your Power Center.

Where Movement Begins

You establish your horse-rider unit the moment you settle into the saddle...but what is it that sets the team in motion? Does movement begin when the horse takes his first step? Does it begin with your first cue to the horse, or some conscious or unconscious activity of your lower leg, seat, or back? Does the horse volunteer to start off, with or without your consent? As a conscious rider and the accepted leader of this horse-rider unit, prepare in both body and mind for your ride before you "cast off." The first few moments often set the tone for the work that will follow.

To prepare, center and increase awareness of your lower spine: the lumbar vertebrae that lie deep within the core of your Power Center. It is here that efficient, balanced movement originates. Deep, abdominal breathing activates the lower spine and brings your focus here. Direct your breath with awareness throughout your body while maintaining your center of gravity making your movements on and off the horse more graceful and composed. With this preparation, you remain more stable, the alignment of your entire body supported by your lower spine and pelvis during any activity.

The heightened awareness of your own movement that yoga practice nurtures can transfer to your riding. During practice, breathe into your Power Center and focus on your lower spine before moving into a pose, consciously preparing for what you are about to do. Visualize your lower spine as a channel that carries and directs energy throughout your body mindfully and sequentially as your breath fuels your movement. With practice, whether moving into or out of a pose, performing a fluid yoga routine, or simply walking with your arms hanging easily by your sides you can create balanced alignment in all your movements as conscious effort becomes more intuitive and kinesthetic.

Follow this same process before beginning your ride. You and your horse will enjoy a stronger connection, moving together more purposefully, rhythmically, and cooperatively. Once in the saddle, breathe deeply, center, and, as your horse awaits your cue, remain mindful of your lower spine as you prepare to activate the horse and set your horse-rider team in motion. From your Power Center, direct prana through your lower spine; energize your torso and limbs and then the horse. Your lower body will sensitively receive and influence his movement as you ride off. When you understand the origins of balanced movement and prepare your mind, body, and horse, you set the tone for a more conscious ride.

SEATED CAMEL

- Chest opens to the sky
- Extend and lift through your spine
- Ground through your seat bones

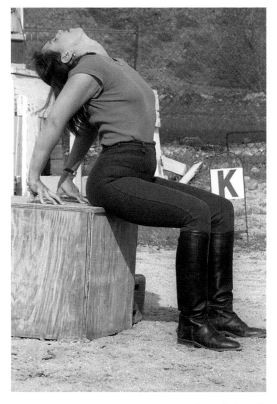

Seated Camel.

RIDER BENEFITS: An exhilarating chest opener and backbend for the rider. Fully stretching the muscles across the chest, this asana counteracts rounded shoulders and a collapsed position. Seated Camel helps increase flexibility in the back and feels fabulous!

1. Begin in any comfortable seated position. Place your hands about eight inches behind your hips, fingers forward (use wrist variation if needed, p. 31).

2. As you inhale, lift and open your chest to the sky, gradually arching your middle and upper back. Drawing your shoulders back and down, gently allow your head to tip back, following the curve of your spine. (If you have any pain or discomfort in your neck, keep your head and eyes forward.) Stay balanced on both seat bones and lift up from your Power Center. With your pelvis anchoring you, allow for a slight pelvic tilt as your lower back flexes to follow the entire spinal arc. Let your arms help support the weight of your torso.

3. Exhale and reaffirm that you are grounded down into the earth as your upper body relaxes further into this backward bend. With each breath, feel the muscles between your ribs expand and your chest open and reach toward the sky; stretch upward from your lower back.

4. Stay here for at least 4 deep and relaxed breaths. When you are ready to release the pose, keep your hands in place to support you while you slowly roll your upper body upward, one vertebra at a time, until you are fully upright. Breathe and center to finish.

COUNTER-POSES: Seated Side Stretch, Half Eagle, Standing Forward Fold

SEATED TWIST

- Extend through your spine
- Shoulders relax down
- Neck and head follow spine

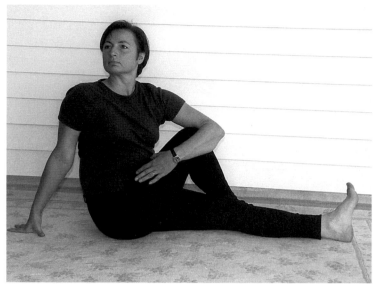

Seated Twist.

Seated Twist – easy variation.

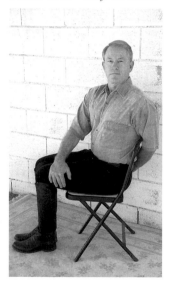

Seated Twist – advanced variation.

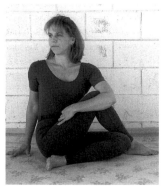

RIDER BENEFITS: Improves elasticity and lateral flexibility of the back, enhancing the rider's ability to receive the horse. Facilitates effective lateral movements on the horse by teaching the rider to stretch and lengthen the spine, rotate the shoulders, and open the chest. Twists are renowned for balancing and aligning the entire spine. Seated Twist is also a rejuvenating and very energizing posture that encourages suppleness through the lower and middle back. Provides a valuable stretch to hips and outer thighs.

1. Begin sitting on the floor with your legs straight out in front of you. Draw your right knee toward your chest and place your right foot against the outside of your left knee.

2. Wrap your left arm around your right knee and hug it into your chest. Inhale deeply and extend tall through your spine.

3. On your next inhalation, stretch your right arm up above you, sweeping your hand around and down to rest on the floor about 8 inches behind your sacrum. Notice how you have already begun to come into the twist to your right. Allow your neck and head to follow the slight rotation of your spine. With every inhalation you take, stretch tall through your entire spine. Push down gently with your back arm to create more lift.

4. On each exhalation, feel your spine rotating from your sacrum all the way to your head like a long spiral. It is particularly important not to force your body in this pose. Rather, use your breathing to allow your body to open at its own pace.

5. Continue stretching up on each inhalation and deepening with each exhalation for 4 breaths or more.

6. Release your hands, slowly unwind and face forward. Rest in Easy Pose for a couple of breaths before proceeding to the other side. To finish, center in Easy Pose.

EASY VARIATION: A simpler version of the Seated Twist can be performed on a chair, mounting block, or bale of hay (shown left).

ADVANCED VARIATION: For an increased twist, fold your extended leg so that your heel comes to meet your opposite hip. Make sure your pelvis and spine can remain upright in this position. If not, you are not yet ready for this variation (shown left).

COUNTER-POSES: Cobbler, Child's Pose

SPINAL FLEX II WITH ROTATION

TIP: This asana is excellent for relieving back discomfort due to tension and stiffness.

RIDER BENEFITS: Improves suppleness of the back. The rotation further increases spinal flexibility and range of motion by fully stretching the muscles that surround the vertebrae. Enhances awareness of initiating movement from the lower spine while maintaining seat bone contact and grounding. Teaches the synchronization of breath and movement, using the breath to direct the rider's motions both in and out of the saddle.

1. Begin in Easy Pose holding your ankles, or sit on the edge of a chair, mounting block, or bale of hay, your hands resting on your knees.

2. Tune in to your breath and feel its natural rhythm. Stay aware of this rhythm; feel how your breath moves through your upper body. Pick a focal point to use throughout.

3. As you inhale, reach forward with your center and chest, rocking onto the front part of your seat bones. Feel the stretch up your spine and out through the top of your head. Let your shoulders drop down and back, opening your chest fully.

4. As you exhale, round your back and rock onto the rear edges of your seat bones. Widen the space between your shoulder blades. Fully stretch the muscles that run along your spine, from your neck to your sacrum.

5. Repeat this sequence, inhaling deeply as you stretch forward and exhaling fully as you rock back. Make your motions as fluid as possible, letting your breath infuse and guide your movements. Continue for at least 8 breaths, more if you like.

6. Begin to make a circle with your spine, rotating your torso and maintaining the same rhythmic breath—inhaling and stretching forward, exhaling and rounding back.

7. Tune in to your seat bones, maintaining contact with the surface you are sitting on. Allow your entire spine to fully enjoy this stretch as you let your upper body flow into wider circles. Listen to your body as you move and let it tell you where you need to stretch deeper or where to go easy. Continue this motion for at least 4-8 breaths, or as long as it feels good to you.

8. Reverse the direction of your circle for an equal number of breaths.

9. To finish, gradually wind down the size of your circle, returning to a still and centered position. Take several soft and easy breaths, close your eyes, and notice how you feel.

Spinal Flex II with Rotation.

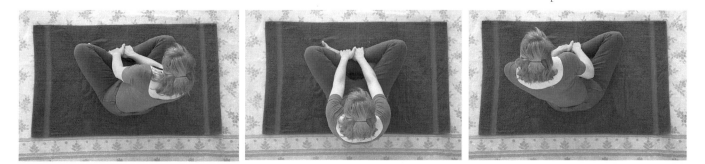

❂

CHAPTER EIGHT

Self-Carriage for the Rider: Upper Body

"...the liberation of the upper part of the body (the head, neck, arms, shoulders, and trunk) produced by the acceptance of gravity in the lower part of the body (legs, feet, knees, and hips) is the origin of lightness, and dancing is its expression." [72]
VANDA SCARAVELLI, *Awakening the Spine*

The rider must develop and refine her own self-carriage before this quality can be expected of the horse.

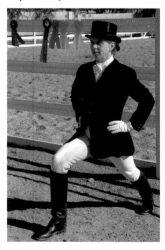

Even though developing the horse's *self-carriage*✳ is a fundamental training objective, the rider's corresponding obligation to self-carry is rarely, if ever, explained by trainers and instructors. It is crucial for the conscious rider to develop and refine self-carriage before this quality can be expected from the horse—and this message should be conveyed early to riding students of any discipline. For the rider to advance toward self-carriage, the upper body must achieve correct balance and sufficient muscle tone and organization to maintain efficient spinal alignment. The following sections address the structures of the torso, with special focus on the head and neck, as well as the arms and hands. Awareness and understanding of the upper body is fundamental to developing rider self-carriage. The asanas of this chapter will help you improve the balance and position of your torso to establish your self-carriage both on and off the horse.

Before beginning this work on the upper body, we highly recommend that you first work through Chapters 6 and 7 to establish the strong foundation within your Sphere of Influence that keeps you centered and grounded, allowing the efficient use of your lower body. When you have confirmed your ability to anchor in the saddle, you will be better able to balance your upper body and stretch freely up through your spine. Following this progressive approach will strengthen your connection with the horse and increase your ability to self-carry.

SECTION 1. Your Torso

A rider's correctly balanced torso is ideally positioned over an upright, supportive pelvis. Because the structures within your Sphere of Influence provide your upper body with a reliable base, the sequential development of an efficient and effective riding position must begin with awareness of your Power Center, the energy source that will ensure your lower body can provide effective support to the torso during all riding activities.

Your spine is an integral supportive structure that extends throughout your torso and includes the delicate area of your neck, an often overlooked spinal component. Spinal misalignment impedes self-carriage and can be caused by a variety of reasons such as injury, poor conformation or postural habits, energy blocks resulting from physical or emotional trauma, or simply sitting or standing for long periods of time. If your posture is neglected, the resulting stress on your spine will not only result in misalignment but can also cause chronic tension through your torso that is often stored in the sensitive head and neck areas, affecting your shoulders and upper back.

We now turn your attention to the interrelated structures of the torso, including your rib cage, chest, shoulders, and upper back. The asanas that follow will assist you in breaking up tension, strengthening and toning your upper body, and establishing the proper alignment and balance of your spine so crucial to achieving self-carriage.

Expansion and Poise

The expansion of your torso is desirable in riding, helping to release tension, reduce rigidity, and eliminate energy blocks. Opening up your torso will enable you to virtually "take up more space" as your body expands to the front, back, left, and right. This becomes possible when your torso is free of tension and your joints flexible, allowing the movement of your breath to foster expansion, rather than creating it forcibly. You also encourage balanced muscle tone throughout your torso by cultivating an open, resilient quality in your upper body. Through correct breathing, your internal supporting structures will naturally and efficiently align without excessive effort. This gentle reorganization of your upper body empowers you to ride with more confidence, awareness, and feeling, broadening your riding experiences and opening you to new possibilities.

Let's examine the structures of your torso to understand how they are involved in developing expansion and poise.

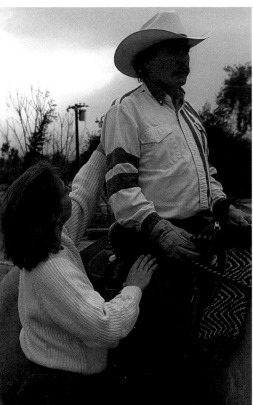

Your spine links your torso and lower body, supporting a vertically aligned position – the balanced seat.

"A weak upper body taxes the lower body by making it work harder to carry and balance a dull torso." [73] JEAN COUCH, *The Runner's Yoga Book*

RIB CAGE

With purposeful breathing, your rib cage expands in all directions. The space this creates throughout your torso quietly assists in releasing tension, encourages your shoulders to soften, stretches your back muscles, lifts your sternum, and opens up your chest.

The *intercostal muscles*✳ span the spaces between your ribs, front to back. When you inhale, these muscles assist the diaphragm in expanding the lungs, like inflated balloons, swelling and lifting your rib cage, raising and expanding your torso to its correct position in your body. When the intercostal muscles relax upon exhaling, the rib cage should ideally remain in this upright position. With practice, you can keep your rib cage effectively placed with the assistance of the upper back muscles. In time, this *relaxed openness* becomes a new habit you bring to all your physical activities, including riding.

The following pranayama facilitates the balanced alignment of your rib cage.

"The rider should sit upright but not stiff, and he should be completely relaxed without slouching. This harmony can only be the result of a long and systematic training of the human body of which ballet dancers give an excellent example." [74] ALOIS PODHAJSKY, *The Complete Training of Horse and Rider*

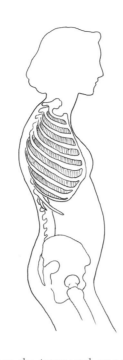

The intercostal muscles help raise the rib cage to its ideal, upright position in your body.

When the intercostal muscles are not engaged, the rib cage collapses, breathing is shallow, and poor posture results.

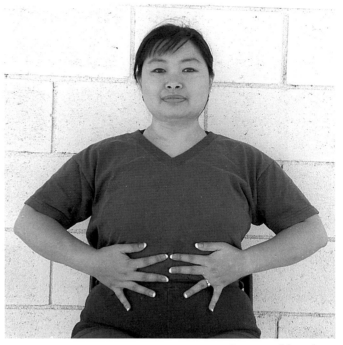

Intercostal breathing.

INTERCOSTAL BREATHING

RIDER BENEFITS: Acquaints the rider with the intercostal muscles. Intercostal Breathing naturally lifts the sternum and helps the rider open the chest. Encourages a more complete use of the lungs and a full expansion of the rib cage. Also assists the rider in efficiently aligning the upper body and elongating through the spine. This is a simple and effective technique to use both in and out of the saddle to remedy poor postural habits such as slouching and collapsing forward.

1. Begin sitting on the edge of a chair, mounting block, or any comfortable surface. Bring your pelvis and spine into balanced alignment as you breathe deeply and rhythmically into your Power Center.

2. Place your palms on either side of your rib cage. Spread your fingers and feel your ribs beneath your hands.

3. With a complete breath, feel the movement of your rib cage as your intercostal muscles expand and contract beneath your hands. Notice how your rib cage naturally lifts within your torso.

4. Release your hands and maintain awareness of this easy, upright, alignment. Continue for at least 8 breaths or until you feel familiar with the movement of your rib cage.

CHEST

"Open your chest!" Riding students commonly hear this directive. Unfortunately, it often prompts a rider to thrust her chest out and up, draw her shoulders back rigidly, and arch her lower back, resulting in swayback and a forced, constricted rearrangement of her body.

Consciously opening your chest begins with your breath and the engagement of your intercostal muscles. You must also strengthen your upper back muscles to help rotate your shoulders back and down. In *Yoga for a New Age*, Bob Smith explains, *"The active muscular work needed to lift the chest is done mainly through the contraction of the upper and middle-back muscles. As these muscles are drawn in toward the spine, the muscles across the chest will passively stretch and expand."* He further emphasizes the importance of *"...rotating the shoulders back and down by drawing the shoulder blades in toward each other, as this brings the upper chest out and allows it to be lifted."*[75]

An expanded chest is a universal equestrian goal, regardless of riding style. Developing both expansion and poise in your upper body will improve your performance on the horse and build both self-carriage and self-confidence, increasing your security in the saddle.

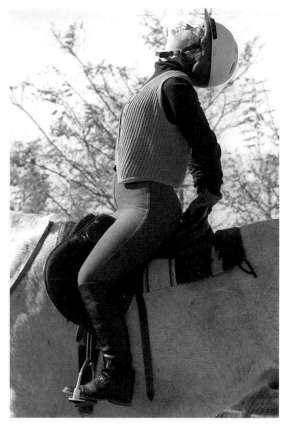

Yoga exercises can help you gradually achieve a balanced, relaxed and expansive posture.

"Confidence is not found in rigidity, but rather in free, relaxed motion."[76] RACHEL SCHAEFFER, *Yoga for Your Spiritual Muscles*

SHOULDERS

As we've learned, to create expansion in the chest, the rider's shoulder joints must release to allow the shoulders to rotate back and down. Adding to the challenge is the barrage of everyday stressors that spark the body's primitive *fight or flight mechanism* ∗ that protectively draws the shoulders up and forward. Under sustained stress, the muscles around the shoulder joints may be almost perpetually contracted, becoming shortened and tight, a storehouse of tension. The shoulders may also become chronically uneven both on and off the horse, with one held higher and closer to the rider's ear than the other.

Shoulder tension and imbalance create substantial energy blocks to riding, preventing the rider from absorbing the movement of the horse. This tension can also be transmitted from the rider, resulting in resistance and anxiety in the horse. Sally Tottle, author of *BodySense*, affirms, *"This ball and socket joint has plenty of potential for movement in all directions, but it is often blocked by tension..."*[77]

When the shoulders become free, the rider increases the capacity to use her arms and hands independently, much like releasing the hip joints allows the rider's legs to work independently of the pelvis. Author and yoga teacher Janet Balaskas explains, *"Your shoulder girdle supports your arms which are connected to it by the round ball and socket joint in the shoulders. This joint is capable of a wide range of movement like the hip joints. Muscles that attach to the entire trunk converge in the shoulder joint rather like the spokes of a wheel. Postures which specifically release the shoulders are very important since imbalance or tightness in the shoulder girdle will affect and disturb the whole body."*[78]

"We usually live on the front part of our bodies and we have developed more on that part, where most of our sensory organs are situated: eyes, nose, mouth, shoulders, hands and chest. Now we have to reverse our attention giving consideration to the back of our body."[79] VANDA SCARAVELLI, Awakening the Spine

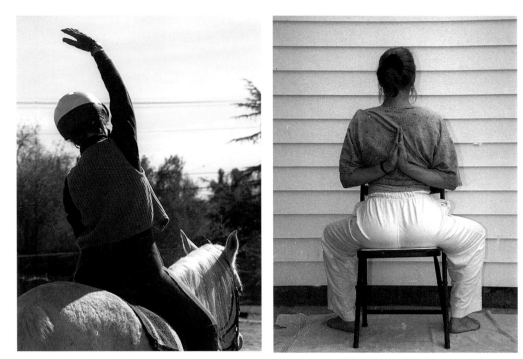

Stretching the upper body loosens the shoulders and frees the arms.

In many ways, yoga teaches us to reverse our attention.

The asanas of this section are fundamental in assisting you with releasing tension through your shoulders, teaching you to let gravity take the weight of your arms down from a shoulder girdle that remains level and balanced.

UPPER BACK

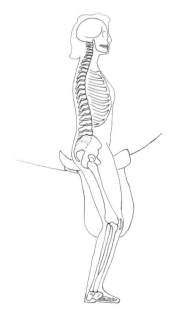

Your skeletal system – a primary determinant of your frame – supports your body. Proper skeletal balance helps define your self-carriage on the horse.

A strong upper back plays a vital role in opening your chest by expanding and lifting your torso. In a torso that collapses forward, the upper back muscles have lengthened and, in order to create expansion and poise in your upper body, they need to be strengthened and realigned by shortening the muscle fibers. Yoga for Equestrians will help you tone and strengthen your upper back muscles to provide better support for your torso as you develop your own self-carriage.

Enhancing awareness of your back contributes to a more balanced alignment and liberates your upper body. We are usually unconscious of our back until it begins to cause us pain or discomfort. As you become more familiar with your back, you learn to trust what you cannot see, gaining a fresh perspective and developing your kinesthetic ability. The asanas that follow encourage the release of energy blocks and tension through your back, allowing gravity to free your upper body, until you can "sit tall" with confidence and poise.

Establishing Your Frame

It is your responsibility to support your position or *frame*✱ with your skeletal structure while sitting astride the horse. Efficient alignment of your bones, the body's supporting structure, coupled with balanced muscle tone are prerequisites to effective equitation and assist the horse in responding correctly and willingly to your aids. Becoming conscious of your frame is a fundamental step on your journey toward Union.

A balanced frame is the basis for establishing your self-carriage, both on and off the horse and is not possible when you attempt to improve alignment or performance by force. Yoga will teach you to guide, encourage, and coax yourself to develop efficient organization of your body.

"But I am Sitting Back!"

In most disciplines, riders are commonly instructed to "sit back" in a riding lesson. Complying with this request is not as easy as it sounds, often involving a battle with the powerful, protective reflex to collapse forward. Lack of confidence or feelings of fear and anxiety may trigger this instinctive reaction while riding. Ironically, this behavior does not protect the rider. On the contrary, it can increase potential risks by disturbing the rider's alignment, preventing a secure connection with the horse.

"But I am sitting back!" is a common student response to an instructor's request; the rider honestly believes she is vertical. What a surprise when the rider actually becomes vertical on the horse and realizes that her body has been providing misleading sensory feedback based on body memory. The rider must learn to override this deceptive sensation and to secure her connection to the horse through grounding and centering, enabling her to align more efficiently and achieve a balanced seat.

The rider's ability to remain in a conscious state of *calm* so that mental focus can be maintained, or quickly recovered, in the event of an upsetting incident on the horse is pivotal to the process of finding the vertical. Avoid panic while on the horse as discord can quickly escalate into a dangerous situation for both horse and rider. Solidify your ability to call on the resources of your Power Center and make your grounding connection *real* so that you can maintain the most stable body position under all circumstances. Another way to ensure calm in the saddle is to cultivate *self-trust*, a quality that is directly related to your level of self-confidence and ability. This will help you maintain a reliably stable, upright position in the saddle, instilling trust in your horse and fostering his ability to trust you.

Yoga practice, especially when performed as a riding warm-up, will nurture a sense of calm that you can bring to your mounted work, enabling you to feel more secure and safe in the saddle. Rather than tipping forward or collapsing your torso, trust your ability and your new instinct to help you find the vertical as you learn how to truly "sit back."

"A balanced seat is the so-called vertical seat, which incidentally appears leaning 'behind the vertical' to some alarmed observers. The term 'vertical' implies a vertical spinal position: the neck of the rider as well as his tailbone are both part of the spine..." [80]
CHARLES DE KUNFFY, *Dressage Questions Answered*

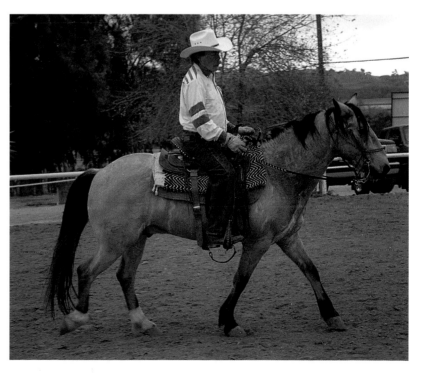

Finding the vertical relies upon your ability to remain in a conscious state of calm to avoid the precarious position caused by collapsing forward on the horse.

CHEST EXPANSION

- Neck is soft
- Extend through your arms

RIDER BENEFITS: Counteracts a rider's collapsed chest and rounded shoulders and releases tension throughout the upper torso. Eliminates energy blocks and increases mobility in the shoulder joints, permitting them to rotate back and down. A strengthening and toning asana for the upper back muscles, it promotes a more upright, vertical alignment, facilitating the rider's self-carriage. Creates openness in the chest, liberating the breath, and encouraging deeper breathing. A beneficial forward bend, Chest Expansion also stretches the hamstrings and encourages the spine to lengthen.

1. Begin in Mountain and step your feet about shoulder width apart.

2. Clasp your hands behind your back and straighten your arms. Open your chest with a deep, intercostal breath and roll your shoulders back and down, reaching your knuckles downward.

3. Fold forward at the hips as you relax your head and neck, letting gravity take the weight of your upper body down.

4. Raise your arms up and away from your lower back as far as you can. Consciously release the muscles of your neck, chest, and shoulders. Bring your shoulder blades closer together as you breathe deeply, expanding your intercostal muscles and the area around your Sphere of Influence. Stay here for at least 4 deep breaths, or longer if you like, releasing tightness with each exhalation.

5. To finish, let your hands come to rest on your lower back, bend your knees slightly, and roll your torso up one vertebra at a time, until you are upright. Release your arms to your sides, and center for a few breaths.

Chest Expansion.

COUNTER-POSES: Half Eagle, Shoulder Circles

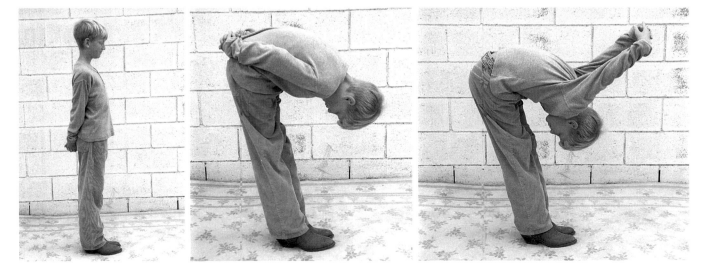

SHOULDER CIRCLES

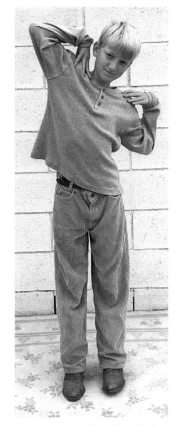

- Big circles with your elbows
- Torso remains upright
- Chest open

RIDER BENEFITS: An easy shoulder loosener that can be done almost anywhere, even in the saddle! This asana is a great upper body warm-up that releases tension in the rider's shoulders and upper back, helping this area move more fluidly. Breaks up energy blocks through the upper body, permitting energy to pass through freely, without resistance. This will strengthen the rider's connection with the horse and is a building block to developing conversational hands and arms, integral elements on this pathway of energy.

1. Begin standing in Mountain or in any comfortable, upright sitting position.

2. Rest your fingers on your shoulders and make a full circle front to back, first with one elbow, then with the other, creating a windmill motion.

3. Continue making circles as you keep your breathing soft and fluid, exploring the range of motion in your shoulders. Continue for at least 8 full rotations, then switch the direction of your circles.

4. To finish, release your arms and return to Mountain. Rest for a moment to enjoy the new energy circulating through your shoulders.

Shoulder Circles.

QUARTER AND HALF DOG

- Lower back and chest sink toward the floor
- Keep feet and legs relaxed

RIDER BENEFITS: Excellent for suppling and releasing tension in the shoulders and upper arms. For riders who are very tight in the shoulder area, these are relatively passive asanas that use gravity to assist in stretching and releasing energy blocks. Both variations stretch and open the chest, while releasing and lengthening the spine.

QUARTER DOG

1. Begin on all fours, hands and knees aligned under your shoulders and hips. Come down onto your elbows, so that they now rest where your hands were.

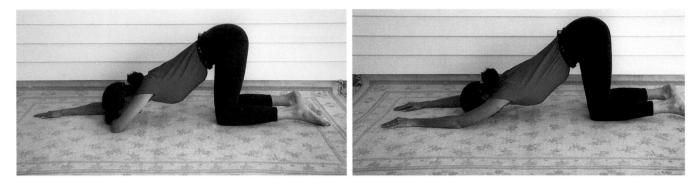

Quarter Dog (left) and Half Dog (right).

2. Bring your left palm to rest under your right elbow.

3. Start walking your right hand forward, letting your shoulders drop down. Keep your thighs perpendicular to the floor. You can scoot your left elbow slightly forward for more extension.

4. Allow your forehead to rest on your left forearm and take 4-8 deep, intercostal breaths in this position. Let your shoulders and upper back release with each exhalation, then feel gravity assist as you release through your whole back.

5. Slowly walk your right hand back, resting on both elbows again. Rest in Child's Pose for a couple of breaths. When you are ready, repeat on the opposite side. For a deeper release, proceed to Half Dog.

HALF DOG

1. Begin on all fours, hands and knees aligned under your shoulders and hips. Come down onto your elbows, so that they now rest where your hands were.

2. Start walking both hands forward, letting your forehead come to rest on the floor as your shoulders drop down. Keep your thighs perpendicular to the floor.

3. Take 4-8 deep, intercostal breaths in this position. Let your shoulders and upper back release with each exhalation, then feel gravity assist as you release through your whole back.

4. To finish, push back into Child's Pose. Rest here for a few breaths.

HALF DOG VARIATION

Here is a variation that's particularly easy to perform in the stable. You will need a pipe corral, barn door, or railing, etc. that is roughly waist-high, for you to hold on to. It must be strong enough to bear your weight.

1. Begin standing in Mountain, approximately an arm's length away from the support that you have chosen.

2. Grasp the rail in front of you with both hands as you bend forward at the hips. Stretch

through your entire spine, including your neck. Hang back from your arms using the rail for support as you stretch your tailbone away from your hands. Take a few breaths here.

3. Flex your feet and rock back on your heels. Take 4-8 breaths in this position. To finish, come back into Mountain.

COUNTER-POSE: Shoulder Circles

SECTION 2. Your Head and Neck

The head and neck are crucial elements of the rider's torso, so strategic that they warrant a section all their own. We will address the important influence of a rider's head and neck and provide the tools to foster their synergetic relationship with the entire spine. Yoga for Equestrians offers helpful techniques to eliminate energy blocks, encourage relaxation, and open up this delicate area, a common storage place for tension.

"If you balance your head correctly, you will discover that you can feel its weight going through your spine right to the seat bones."[81] SALLY SWIFT, Centered Riding

Atlas and Axis

Your neck contains an integral section of your spine, the cervical vertebrae. The cervical vertebrae must be mindfully included when establishing balanced spinal alignment both on and off the horse. Many riders inadvertently overlook their necks when attempting to "sit tall" or find the vertical, often resulting in an accentuated neck curve and the misalignment of the cervical vertebrae.

The cervical curve is the smallest of the natural curves of your spine. Poor postural habits like rounded shoulders, a collapsed chest, or an imbalanced head increase the curvature of your cervical spine. This curvature impacts the first two cervical vertebrae, the *atlas*✳ and *axis*✳.

In understanding the importance of these vertebrae, we turn to Gray's Anatomy: *"The first cervical vertebra is named the atlas because it supports the globe of the head."*[82] The atlas, named after a Titan in Greek mythology who was forced by the gods to bear the weight of the world on his shoulders is jointed and articulates with the second cervical vertebra, called the axis *"because it forms the pivot upon which the first vertebra, carrying the head, rotates."*[83] Together, the atlas and axis permit the rotation and nodding movements of your head so it is crucial that they are free from muscular tension that restricts their function.

Because many modern-day riders are like Atlas, carrying the weight of *their* world on their shoulders, strain throughout the upper torso is commonplace. If tension becomes lodged at the top of the spine where the cervical vertebrae meet the skull, an excessive curve in the neck results. Bob Smith explains, *"The greatest curve in the neck generally occurs where the top two vertebrae of the neck and the back of the skull meet. Many people hold a large amount of tension at the top of the neck because of excess curvature here."*[84]

To release tension in the sensitive atlas-axis area, direct your breath between

Alignment of the head and cervical vertebrae.

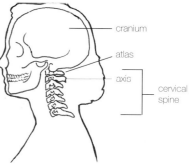

these vertebrae and your head to increase space and allow energy to flow freely. Making these adjustments through yoga practice increases awareness of your cervical vertebrae and gently improves the alignment of your neck. Consciously establishing better postural habits will enhance your self-carriage on the horse.

Allowing Gravity

"Gravity is like a magnet attracting us to the earth, but this attraction is not limited to pulling us down, it also allows us to stretch in the opposite direction towards the sky."[85]
VANDA SCARAVELLI,
Awakening the Spine

If your frame is not efficiently supported by the skeletal system, your muscles work overtime attempting to keep your body upright and your head balanced. Both inactivity and repetitive activity can cause the natural curves throughout your spine to become misaligned, which severely taxes the muscles of your upper back, neck, and shoulders. Head and neck stiffness are common symptoms of chronic muscular stress.

Because the neck muscles extend into your shoulders and upper back, these areas can also store tension, obstructing the flow of energy and movement. Continual contraction of the muscles of your neck and back can result in common rider problems such as strained muscles, upper body resistance to the horse's movement, inflexible shoulder joints and spine, frequent headaches, and a high center of gravity. Judith Lasater, author of *Relax and Renew*, explains, *"This tension is actually your body's attempt to hold itself upright in a difficult, distorted position. The muscles of the neck and shoulders become knotted and fatigued as they try to resist gravity."[86]*

Yoga for Equestrians enhances your ability to release tension through gentle stretching, as well as partial inversions of the head that use gravity to facilitate release. In order to allow gravity to help you achieve ideal balance of head, neck, and spine, it is imperative that you first establish your foundation: the upright alignment of your pelvis and a secure grounding connection through your lower body.

Allow gravity to take the weight of your head and gently release your neck muscles.

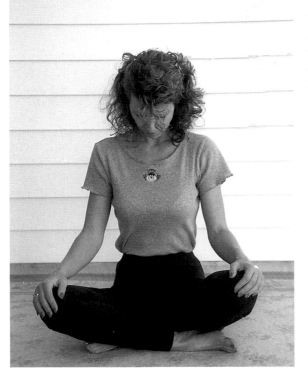

Once you are grounded, direct your breath to move prana through your spine, one vertebra at a time, to establish upright alignment and the balance of your head. Reduce excessive muscular effort by letting gravity help free and release your muscles. With your frame efficiently organized and supported and your center of gravity in place, allow the back of your neck to extend and lengthen even further, enjoying the sensation of your head "floating" upward, like a helium balloon tethered by a securely anchored line.

Ideal Balance

The ability of a rider to self-carry relies on the stabilizing quality of the Sphere of Influence and correct alignment of the spine, topped with a softly balanced head. The seat bones provide a strong base of support and are directly involved in stabilizing the rider's head. Essentially, a rider's effective alignment on the horse begins with the seat bones and extends all the way up the spine to the head.

The substantial weight of your head can significantly influence your entire balance and position on the horse. Ideally, your head should be balanced lightly atop your spine, resting evenly above your neck, where your first cervical vertebra, the atlas, is jointed with your cranium. Riders commonly experience a lack of balance in the head, generally resulting from weakness in the supporting structures below. A rider who allows her head to tip off balance from the neck in any direction, and at any angle, exerts a burdensome pressure on the uppermost cervical vertebrae and the musculature of the neck, shoulders, and upper back.

Performing activities with your head tipped back or your arms above your head for prolonged periods of time can compact the discs between the vertebrae, causing irritation to the nerves that run through the cervical spine. Familiar horse-related activities like grooming, braiding or clipping, removing cobwebs with a broom, painting the ceiling of your tack room, etc., involve tipping your head backward for extended periods and may contribute to strained muscles and compression in the cervical vertebrae. A head carried either forward or down can result in undue strain on the supportive muscles of the neck, shoulders, and upper back, often contributing to headaches, muscle soreness, and spinal misalignment.

If your head is positioned in front of your center of gravity when riding, its weight often draws your shoulders, arms, and upper back forward, creating an unstable and misaligned position in the saddle. An unbalanced head can also cause loss of balance in the horse. For example, if your head drops forward, you may inadvertently shift your body weight over the horse's shoulders, greatly affecting his performance. Some horses may fall on the forehand, stumble, or wobble underneath you; others begin to rush, increasing speed as they attempt to "catch up" with your forward weight shift and misplaced center of gravity; others may slow down, or stop completely, offering you an opportunity to rebalance and organize your position. As you can see, an unbalanced head position can greatly interfere with your riding performance and prevent self-carriage in both horse and rider.

An often overlooked aspect of the rider's head is the face. Chronic tension can result in a locked jaw, clenched teeth, and furrowed brow, as well as eye strain, headaches, and sinus problems. Remedies for facial tension include pranayama, meditation, conscious relaxation, stretching, and massage, but perhaps the easiest remedy is a smile! Smiling, enjoying yourself, having more fun, and letting go of self-criticism and judgment will all ultimately contribute to relaxing the intricate muscles of your face.

The following visualization ignites an energy flow from deep within your Power Center that surges up through your spine and out the top of your head, helping you experience ideal balance.

UNMOUNTED VISUALIZATION: Skyward Energy Flow

In Easy Pose, close your eyes and breathe deeply, flooding your Sphere of Influence with your breath. Ground firmly into the surface below you. Balance evenly on your seat bones and begin to direct prana with your breath up through your spine from your Power Center. Take your awareness up slowly, vertebra by vertebra. With every inhalation, feel your torso lengthen as your spine aligns vertically. Breathe space in between each vertebra. With every exhalation, solidify the grounding through your seat bones and release tension with your breath.

See or feel the prana bringing a vibration of color, light, or a tingling sensation up

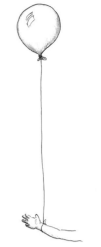

Imagine your head floating up from your spine like a balloon tethered by a thin line.

"Unless the head sits straight on top of the neck, an imbalance of energy will be created."[87] BOB SMITH, *Yoga for a New Age.*

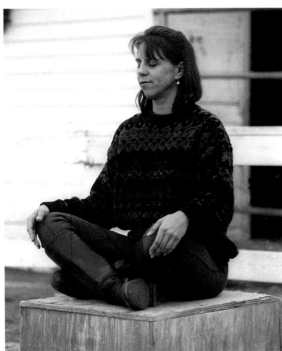

Direct your breath up your spine, creating an energy pathway that connects you to the sky above.

through your spine until it arrives at the base of your skull. Visualize a gap here, creating more space between the atlas and your head. Let prana bridge this gap and continue to flow up the back of your head. Feel the energy circulate throughout your scalp and face, relaxing your cheeks, eyelids, and jaw.

Ensure that the vertebrae in your neck are straight by gently extending the back of your head upward. Feel the prana continue to spread throughout your scalp and emit outward through the top of your head into the sky or the space above you. Experience the sensation of lightness as your neck stretches up, releasing your head to balance effortlessly on your neck.

Now, connect yourself to what is above as you draw energy from the sky into your body through the top of your head; channel it down your spine to replenish your Power Center, which amplifies that energy. Now circulate it back up through your body again, out through top of your head. Creating this energy pathway connects you to what is above, much like grounding connects you to what is below. Experience this resonant connection with both earth and sky. Feel your spine as a connecting link between the two directions. Breathe deeply here.

When you are finished, slowly open your eyes knowing that you can reconnect at any time to this energy flow.

The following asanas will help you release head, neck, and torso tension, fostering the ideal balance and alignment necessary for your self-carriage on and off the horse.

HORSESHOE STRETCH

- Shoulders relax down
- Relax your jaw
- Keep your spine aligned

RIDER BENEFITS: This is a gentle, deep stretch for the muscles along the back and sides of the rider's neck. Done slowly and with awareness, it helps the rider target specific areas of tightness in the neck by loosening the muscles, increasing flexibility of the cervical spine. This relaxing stretch helps create space between the atlas and axis vertebrae and the head, breaking up energy blocks through this area and enhancing the rider's ability to carry the head lightly, with more poise.

1. Begin in a comfortable sitting position. Center and ground, as you align vertically through your upper body. Breathe intercostally, expanding your chest and relaxing your shoulders.

2. Gently drop your head forward and down, giving in to gravity. Maintain the upright and relaxed alignment of your torso and imagine a heavy velvet robe, or a pair of gentle hands resting on your shoulders, encouraging them to drop down, away from your ears. Breathe deeply.

3. Roll your head slowly toward your left shoulder, allowing gravity to minimize the muscular effort. Pause for a breath and feel the stretch. Release tension as you exhale.

4. Let your head slowly roll back to center and over to your right shoulder, making a horseshoe-shaped arc. Check your shoulders to ensure they are still relaxed down and level.

5. Repeat 4-8 sets, maintaining deep fluid breathing. Let go of trying and allow gravity to encourage the stretch as you release through your neck and shoulder muscles.

6. To finish, bring your head back to center. Breathe normally.

Horseshoe Stretch.

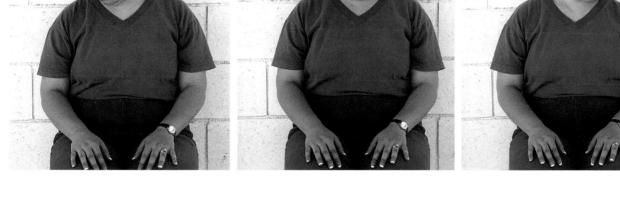

BENT WILLOW

- Keep torso upright
- Shoulders are relaxed

RIDER BENEFITS: This is an excellent asana for riders who carry stress in their upper shoulders and their neck. It provides a deep release for the muscles and ligaments of this area, helping to break up energy blocks. This gentle stretch can enhance flexibility in the rider's neck, increasing range of motion.

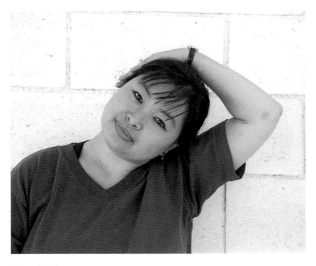

Bent Willow.

1. Begin with Horseshoe Stretch, then let your head roll over to your right shoulder and remain.

2. Place the palm of your right hand flat on your head, above your ear. Let gravity take the weight of your head toward your shoulder. Take care that you don't collapse your upper body—stay light and extended through your spine and relax your shoulders.

3. Breathe deeply here, bringing in relaxation as you inhale and releasing all tension as you exhale. Stay here as long as you wish.

4. Slowly roll your head to the left and repeat.

5. To finish, return to Horseshoe Stretch, completing 2-4 sets, then bring your head back to center. Breathe normally.

HARE

- Lift out of your shoulders
- Legs stay relaxed

RIDER BENEFITS: Provides an intense and deep stretch for the back of the neck, extending into the upper and middle back, and effectively breaks up tension throughout this entire area. This asana releases compression in the cervical vertebrae, helping to counteract the effects of bad postural habits that may have compacted this portion of the spine. Being a partially inverted pose, Hare is helpful in clearing the mind and enhancing alertness.

Hare.

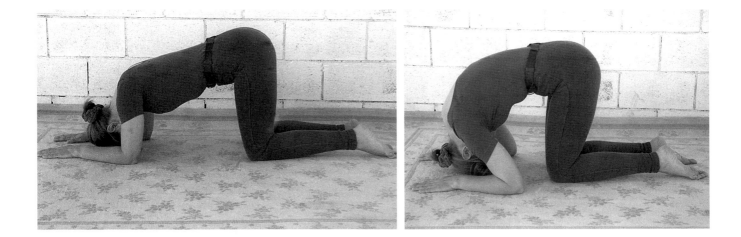

TIP: Before practicing Hare, please review the guidelines for inverted poses on p. 30.

1. Begin on all fours, hands and knees aligned underneath your shoulders and hips. Come down onto your elbows, placing them where your hands were.

2. Rest the top of your head on the floor between your elbows.

3. With awareness, gradually begin walking your knees toward your elbows. Round your upper spine, feeling a stretch to the your neck and upper back. Let your arms support you, keeping weight off of your head and neck. Stretch out of your shoulders, lengthening them down away from your ears.

4. Find the degree of stretch that is right for you, then breathe deeply in that position for at least 4 breaths.

5. To finish, slowly move back into Child's Pose for several breaths before coming to an upright position.

COUNTER-POSES: Seated Camel, Horseshoe Stretch, Bent Willow

STANDING FORWARD FOLD

- Release at the hip
- Shoulder blades relax down

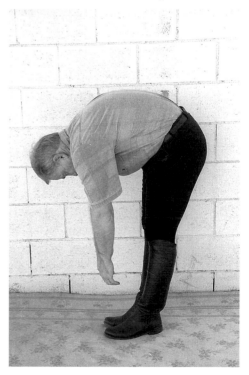

Standing Forward Fold.

RIDER BENEFITS: This simple asana uses gravity to assist in releasing the vertebrae. Helps break up muscle tension and releases compaction through the neck. Creates space between the atlas vertebra and the head and releases the shoulder joints. As gravity takes the weight of the upper body, the rider's hamstrings also receive a deep, passive stretch.

1. Begin in Mountain. Soften your knees and let your breathing be relaxed and fluid.

2. Gently drop your chin toward your chest. Leading with your head, let gravity take your upper body down, one vertebra at a time, as far as you can. Let your arms hang down loosely.

3. Breathe deeply and let gravity completely take the weight of your upper body. Consciously relax and release all the muscles along your back, paying particular attention to your neck and shoulders. Let your head dangle freely as tension flows out with each exhalation. Stay here for 8 deep breaths or longer.

4. Come out of the pose the same way you went in, rolling up slowly, one vertebra at a time, until you are upright again. Breathe and center before moving on.

SECTION 3. Conversational Hands and Relaxed Arms

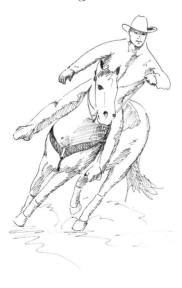

Strive to develop educated hands that sensitively communicate with the horse.

A rider's hands can be taught to deliver subtle signals that "converse" with the horse and regulate the flow of forward energy that travels from the hindquarters through the rider's arms to the bridle. Conversational hands require dexterous fingers, wrists, elbows, and shoulders. Soft and flexible joints allow a rider's hands to more sensitively and effectively communicate with the horse.

Ineffective or counterproductive use of the hands and arms is another symptom of a weak rider foundation. In order to make effective corrections in your upper body, it is essential that your base of support be secure first. Again, we strongly encourage you to achieve the ability to center and ground yourself, deepen your connection to the horse, and consciously support your body with the stabilizing structures of your Sphere of Influence and spine before focusing on your hands and arms.

Increasing Forward Energy Flow

Riding activities that involve either high speed or dynamic movement require an enhanced ability to absorb and channel energy freely through your upper body to allow you to regulate and direct the horse's energy.

In order to achieve self-carriage, the horse's movement must flow freely through your upper body. Blocked energy or stiffness in the upper body can cause unintentional movement of your arms and hands. The resulting misuse of the reins is typically responsible for creating resistances or vices and can injure or desensitize the horse's sensitive mouth. When upper body tension is released, your torso becomes better able to channel and absorb movement and forward energy while riding, increasing comfort and efficiency for both horse and rider.

The **shoulder joints,** important connecting structures of the torso, are pivotal to rider self-carriage and the proper use of arms and hands. Correct position and balance on the horse relies on free shoulder joints. The rider must strive to increase the range of motion in the shoulders as a crucial preliminary step to achieving independent hands.

Your **upper arms** should hang from the shoulder joints in a relaxed manner, letting gravity take them downward. If your upper arms extend rigidly in front of your body from locked shoulder joints, they draw your entire torso forward, overloading the horse's forehand and disturbing the alignment and balance of your horse-rider pair. A balanced equestrian does not overuse the biceps or triceps muscles while riding. Doing so may lead to a pulling match with the horse, one that most riders can never win and that usually results in the rider bracing her shoulders against the horse. Such heavy handling can cause the horse to lean on the rein or balance off the rein during either sustained movement or transitions, creating a cycle of imbalance that must be corrected. The rider must do less with these muscles and learn to relax and release her arms to gravity.

The **elbow joint** is an important hinge. When free and elastic, this joint allows the rider's forearm to become an extension of the rein, increasing the rider's ability to communicate through the hands. The elbow joint must be bent, creating an angle no less than 90 degrees (a more open elbow creates an angle slightly greater than 90 degrees). It is important that this bend does not become *fixed*. Rather, the elbow joint must be permitted to fluidly adjust in response to the horse's movements, channeling forward energy and absorbing concussive movements as in the trot, during which the elbow acts much like a spring to prevent the hands from bouncing.

Your elbow is a connecting link along the path of energy that courses through your horse-rider team and, if it becomes rigid and locked, it breaks the flow. Stiffness in the elbow joints and shoulders may cause the rider's arms to swing awkwardly from the shoulder joints. It is important to develop an elastic quality in your elbow, to better follow the movement of the horse's head and neck and encourage energy to flow through.

In riding styles such as dressage and English equitation where contact is established by creating a straight line with the rider's forearm and rein from elbow to bit, the rider's **forearm** becomes an extension of the rein. In Western equitation, the forearm of the reining hand must be softly supported by supple joints in the elbow, wrist, and shoulders, which absorb movement and appear quiet and still. The forearm should never weigh down the rein; the rider's fingers and wrists should ideally communicate deft and subtle cues to the horse on a soft, relaxed rein. Although the interconnected muscles of the forearms, wrists, and hands may tighten unconsciously, a rider must learn to consciously release this tension to prevent its transference through their fingers to the bit.

The rider's **wrists** should be straight, not crooked, curved, bent, or flat. These delicate areas must remain a channel for forward energy and movement, and must not take responsibility for holding the reins, which is the job of your fingers and hands. Often, the rider's wrists are overly used to "supple" the rein, curling incorrectly in an attempt to soften the horse's jaw. It is important to avoid repetitive movements of the wrist in riding, as Carpal Tunnel Syndrome and other related problems may result. Learn to keep your wrists soft, straight, and open to channel energy forward into your hands and fingers.

Your **fingers** should wrap around the reins in a soft but firm fist. They create an elastic connection to the horse's mouth, a feeling that takes a considerable amount of time to develop. That is why it is so important to ride on the longe line as often as you can, to increase the stability of your seat and ensure optimal alignment. These fundamental skills will lead to a feeling of connection with the horse's mouth. Mounted exercises for the upper body (such as Yoga in the Saddle, see Chapter 10), that are performed on the longe line, will strengthen the security of your seat and help release your hands from incorrectly "hanging on." A firm foundation and a secure seat will allow you to then converse lightly and sensitively with your fingers.

When your arms are sufficiently suppled and toned, yet relaxed and yielding, you experience a heightened flow of forward energy through these channels. You can direct this flow with your breath, allowing prana from the horse to surge forward through your arms and out toward his head and neck. It is an exhilarating feeling that lightens and refines your communication with the horse and, because it is energetic, your connection will also become subtly stronger, bringing you closer to Union.

Independent Hands

Your hands are important communication aids that convey your intentions and directions to the horse via the reins. It is important that your hands learn how to *separate* or *disengage* from both your movement and the horse's motion, as they do when holding a drink in a moving car—the bumpier the ride, the more stable your hands must remain lest you

Activate and extend the lines of energy through your arms and into the bridle.

"Contact...refers to every aspect of exchange that takes place between the horse and rider. It implies a mutual relationship, based on reciprocity. It ends up being the most observable in the rider's hands, but the hands are only a manifestation of the entire position. If the rider's hands, and thus the contact, is poor, it is because his/her fundamental position is not sufficiently developed."[88] SHERRY L. ACKERMAN, *Dressage in the Fourth Dimension*

end up wearing your drink! To keep you dry, the rest of your body absorbs the motion, especially the joints of your arms. In the saddle, the joints of your arms act as shock absorbers, dispersing the horse's movements much like shocks on a car provide a smoother ride over the bumps.

Locked joints block absorption of the horse's movement and transmit tension through your arms to the horse, rather than allowing motion to pass through. This can lead to conflicting and unintentional rein cues, over-active hands, and excessive pressure on the horse's mouth. Backward pressure on the bit can distort the horse's shape into a hollow, tense, or shortened frame.

Clumsy rein handling can be considered a form of painful abuse of the horse. The unskilled rider who relies on the reins for balance is often an unwitting culprit. The patient horse that tolerates a rider's bouncing hand movements may soon become "hard-mouthed" or desensitized. This horse may also mentally shut down and ignore the rider, unable to distinguish between rein aids and the constant movement of the rider's hands.

Educated, conversational hands regulate the forward flow of energy like a valve, encouraging it during upward transitions and the medium and extended gaits; restraining it during downward transitions and the collected and slower gaits like the Western jog. The potential conversation between the rider's hands and the horse's mouth is so complex that the hands must achieve their own independent dynamic stillness. Although ideal hands appear to remain in one place, they are not dull or unmoving. The rider's hands make frequent adjustments that are so minute that they may be invisible to on-lookers, yet these quiet cues are received by the horse's highly sensitive mouth and head through the action of the bit and bridle.

Developing independence of your hands on the horse is a complex task. Realize that achieving this goal will take practice and discipline. If you suspect that you are misusing your hands, honor the horse by gaining stability and finer control first in an unmounted setting or on the longe line. Use yoga practice to facilitate the release of tension through your arms and hands, to keep your joints soft and the energy channels open to establish a better *feel*. The asanas that follow address upper body issues, and improve your ability to ride the horse with light, independent, conversational hands.

Remember, riders...as you journey, the final stage to achieving Union with the horse is truly in your hands.

SWINGING TWIST

- Knees stay soft and slightly bent
- Ground through your feet

RIDER BENEFITS: For riders who are restricted through their upper body, this asana is a perfect remedy. Swinging Twist releases tension and stiffness while encouraging freedom of movement through the hands, arms, and shoulders with gentle loosening and unconstrained movement. It is also beneficial for keeping the joints of the legs supple, able to accommodate the motion of the upper body.

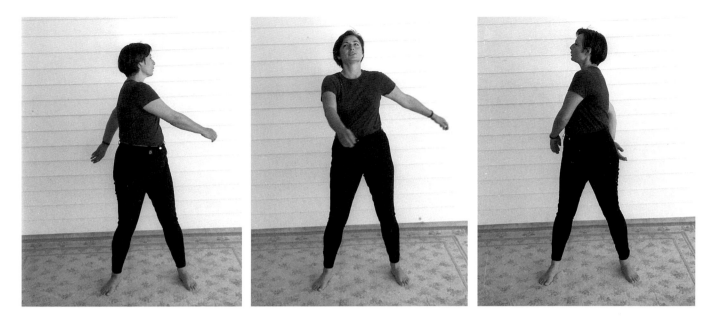

Swinging Twist.

CAUTION: If you have knee problems, twist more from your hips, keeping your legs and pelvis stable to prevent torquing your knees.

1. Begin standing with your feet about shoulder width apart or wider, toes pointed forward; knees supple and slightly bent. Breathe deeply.

2. Imagine you are a rag doll. Slowly twist left, then right, letting your arms swing loosely. Continue twisting from side to side, gradually increasing the tempo.

3. Let your breathing soften your body and fuel your movement. Get your whole body into the twist: shoulders, waist, and hips. Slightly bend each knee while twisting, bringing your legs into the motion as well. Continue as long as your body enjoys it!

4. To finish, wind down gradually, coming back to center. Breathe fully into your body, feeling relaxed and alive!

HALF EAGLE

- Arms extend upward
- Shoulders relax down

RIDER BENEFITS: Loosens the elbow and shoulder joints, bringing a deep stretch through the muscles and ligaments of the upper torso. Also provides isometric strengthening of forearms, wrists, and hands. Ideal for riders who carry tension through their upper or middle back, Half Eagle releases the space between the shoulder blades and breaks up energy blocks.

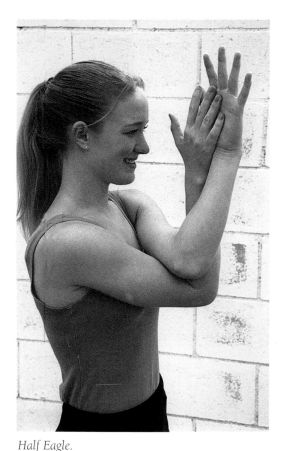

Half Eagle.

1. Begin in a comfortable seated or standing position. Take a few deep, intercostal breaths, growing tall and light through your upper body. Choose a focal point in front of you.

2. Bring your right arm in front of you, bending your elbow. Point your forearm straight up with a flat palm facing left.

3. Wrap your left arm under your right elbow, bringing it straight up on the right side, palm facing right.

4. Bring the fingers of your left hand to rest on the palm of your right hand. If this is a difficult reach for you, try linking a finger with your thumb. Adjust the degree of stretch by either lowering or raising your elbows.

5. Gaze straight ahead, past your arms and breathe deeply into your Power Center. Direct your breath into the space between your shoulder blades, consciously releasing tension there with each exhalation. Hold for at least 4 deep breaths. Gradually work your way up to 8 breaths or more.

6. Release your arms slowly and consciously, stretching them in any way that feels good. Reverse your arm position and repeat.

COUNTER-POSES: Chest Expansion, Shoulder Circles, Cow's Face

Cow's Face.

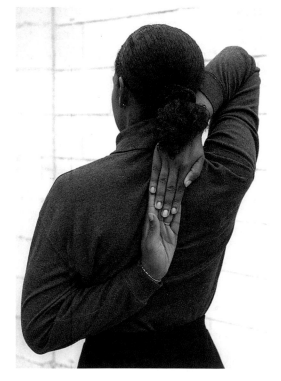

COW'S FACE

- Arm stays close to ear
- Keep head upright

RIDER BENEFITS: Dissolves tension and increases range of motion in the rider's upper back, shoulders, and elbows, supporting the independent use of the rider's arms. This asana encourages the spine to align, the chest to open, and shoulders to draw back. Counteracts the common rider habit of rounding the back and collapsing forward. Also increases breathing capacity.

TIP: For Step 3, use readily available items such as a lead rope, crop, towel, riding glove, etc., as props.

1. Begin in a comfortable seated or standing position. Lengthen through your upper body, open your chest, and bring your shoulders back and down. Choose a focal point in front of you.

2. Reach behind your back with your left arm, placing your left hand as high up on your spine as you can.

3. With a deep inhalation, stretch your right arm straight up over your head. Bend your elbow and reach down toward the center of your back. Can your hands touch each other? If so, hook your fingers or grasp hands, depending on your level of flexibility. If not, use a prop to bridge the gap.

4. Gently move your hands closer together to increase the stretch. Listen closely to your body and *respect your edges*. Remember to breathe!

5. Gaze straight ahead and take several intercostal breaths to open and lift your chest. Reaching your elbows straight up and down; relax your shoulders as much as you can to help them release and open. With each breath, lighten, release, and expand! Hold for at least 4 deep breaths. Gradually work your way up to 8 breaths or more.

6. Come out of this pose slowly and consciously. Shake out your arms and stretch in any way that feels good to you. Repeat on the opposite side, stretch and shake out again. Now, breathe and center.

COUNTER-POSES: Shoulder Circles, Horseshoe Stretch, Half Eagle, Child's Pose

REVERSE NAMASTE

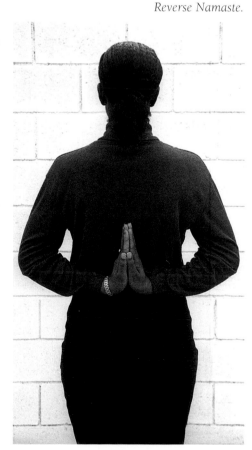

Reverse Namaste.

Namaste (pronounced "Nah-Mah-Stay") is a Sanskrit word that means "the spirit in me honors the spirit in you."

• Look straight ahead
• Shoulders stay relaxed

RIDER BENEFITS: Stretches the muscles and tendons spanning the arms and upper chest, allowing the rider's arms to move more independently of the torso when in the saddle. Encourages the rider's shoulders to come back and the chest to open, facilitating deeper and more expansive breathing.

TIP: If you have Carpal Tunnel Syndrome, wrist injuries, or if Reverse Namaste is too challenging, try Hand/Elbow Clasp as a variation.

1. Begin in a comfortable sitting or standing position. Take a few deep intercostal breaths to help you lengthen and expand through your upper body. Choose a focal point in front of you.

2. Reach both hands behind your lower back, palms facing. With your fingers pointed up and tips touching, gradually bring your palms as close together as you can. Stretch your shoulders back and down as you

open and expand your chest, finding your place in the pose. Stretch tall and light for at least 4 deep breaths, gradually working up to 8 breaths or more.

3. To finish, release your hands and stretch out your arms.

COUNTER-POSES: Shoulder Circles, Half Eagle

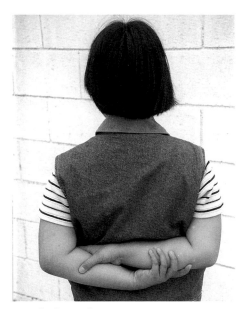

Hand/Elbow Clasp.

HAND/ELBOW CLASP

RIDER BENEFITS: A less challenging variation and often a preliminary step to performing Reverse Namaste; offers similar benefits.

1. Repeat Step 1, above.

2. Reach both hands behind your back, and clasp your wrists. Breathe deeply, bringing your shoulders back and down away from your ears.

3. Walk your fingers toward your elbows. With awareness, find your place in the pose. Expand your chest and draw your shoulders back and down. Breathe and relax into this position for at least 4 deep breaths. Gradually work your way up to 8 breaths or more.

4. Slowly release and gently stretch out your arms. Breathe and center before moving on.

PART IV

The Journey Continues

"We must find ways to soar to unseen dimensions.
That flight begins with our imaginations. We must reach beyond the
possible to the impossible, and touch the untouchable."[89]
ADELE VON RÜST AND MARLENA DEBORAH MCCORMICK, PH.D.,
Horse Sense and the Human Heart

CHAPTER NINE

Establishing Your Practice

EVERY RIDER (and her horse) can benefit from an effective and convenient rider warm-up before mounting. Because of its balanced nature, yoga practice is ideal in preparing you for both the physical and mental connection you seek with the horse. A yoga warm-up will help you become more supple, balanced, and efficient in the saddle. The horse also benefits from the enhanced levels of relaxation, focus, and flexibility yoga brings to your riding. Increased body awareness furthers effective communication with the horse, making your work together more synchronized and pleasurable.

After riding, most equestrians will take time to cool down their horses appropriately, often overlooking their similar need. To remedy this, the yoga cool-down practices we provide will help you wind down from your ride. They gradually bring down your heart rate and slowly cool your muscles, reducing stress on your body and helping to prevent soreness after a ride.

The Yoga Routines

The routines we provide vary in focus and character. Gentle, slow, and relaxing routines are balanced by more invigorating and dynamic ones. Choose the one that best suits your riding goals and meets your energy level. Alternate between practices as your needs change.

Each routine offers various durations to choose from. If you are pressed for time or feel anxious to mount up and ride, choose the shorter routines. When you have the time, opt for a more complete practice. Adjust your pace as you go, using what works best for you. We do recommend that you establish a consistent habit of warming up before you ride. You will find that even a *five minute* yoga warm-up will benefit both you and the horse!

The following routines serve as general outlines to help you integrate Yoga for Equestrians into your riding program. Once you have become familiar and comfortable with yoga, you can tailor your practice to suit your individual needs. (Refer back to Chapter 3 to help you balance your practice and see Appendix 4 for a guide to asanas and pranayama.)

About Warming Up

Warming up with yoga can help you feel more energetic and connected to the horse. An important aim of stretching and warming up, for riders or *anyone* preparing to engage in a physical activity, is to avoid injury by suppling your body. Yoga helps to increase flexibility and range of motion in the joints and muscles you will use in riding. Warming up provides your body the opportunity to stretch and become more elastic and, therefore, better able to perform without tension or strain.

TIP: Should you ever feel "spacey," sleepy, or *too* relaxed after your practice, we recommend that you do one or several of the following before mounting the horse so that you are alert and bright for your ride:

DEFINITELY DO:

- Arm Raise with Breath, p. 46

- Breath of Joy, p. 47-48

ADD IF NECESSARY:

- Swinging Twist, p. 138-139

- Standing Forward Fold, p. 135

SECTION 1. Yoga Warm-Ups

These warm-ups incorporate *supine*✱ poses and are designed to be done at home, work, or wherever you have a comfortable floor space. Weather permitting, take a mat, towel, or horse blanket outside to a comfortable spot, and enjoy the outdoors! "Rise and Shine" is low key, letting you ease gently into your day, whereas "Changing Hats" is designed for making the transition from work or other daily activities to riding.

"RISE and SHINE"—Start the Flow

This practice is a great way to start your day. Your muscles are usually the least flexible in the morning, so these asanas will gently encourage your body to wake up and begin to stretch. Move with awareness and sensitivity, breathing deeply and slowly as you practice. If you feel particularly stiff or cold, you may want to take a hot shower, turn the heat up a notch, or put on an extra layer of clothing to help warm your muscles before your practice.

REFLECTIONS: *Bring in fresh, new energy with each breath during this practice. Even if it's cloudy outside, imagine breathing in bright rays of sunlight or a fresh breeze. With each exhalation, imagine your body opening gradually to the day; feel your muscles begin to lengthen and soften. Focus on what feels good to your body. Put on some uplifting music and feel the energy flow!*

TAKE FIVE (5 MINUTES)
- Breathe Into Your Back
- Cat Stretch
- Breath of Joy

SHORT PRACTICE (10 MINUTES)
- Breathe Into Your Back
- Cat Stretch
- Happy Baby
- Bridge
- Breath of Joy

MEDIUM PRACTICE (15-20 MINUTES)
- Breathe Into Your Back
- Cat Stretch
- Half Dog
- Hare
- Bridge
- Toe Touch
- Happy Baby
- Breath of Joy
- Arm Raise with Breath

"Rise and Shine" – medium practice.

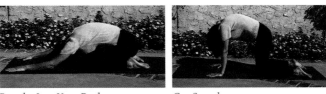

Breathe Into Your Back   *Cat Stretch*   *Half Dog*

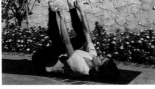

Hare   *Bridge*   *Toe Touch*

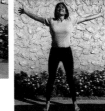

Happy Baby

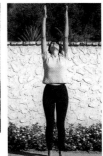

Breath of Joy

Arm Raise with Breath

This is a good opportunity to add:
- Meditation
- Visualization
- Mental rehearsal of your ride

"CHANGING HATS"—A Transition

This practice provides a great way to make the transition from your daily activities to riding. For instance, you may be coming from a job or activity that requires you to sit or stand for long periods, resulting in tightness in your back, legs, and shoulders. Or you may have dealt with a lot of stress during the day and find it challenging to "change hats" from the concerns of work to the more enjoyable activity of riding. The following asanas will take you nicely through this type of transition.

We include pranayama to calm and focus your mind, asanas to stretch muscles neglected during the day, and then combine both to help invigorate body and mind and bring in fresh energy so you can fully enjoy your favorite activity!

REFLECTIONS: *Release tension every time you exhale; bring in rejuvenating energy with each inhalation. Anytime your mind begins to wander, gently lead it back to what your body is doing. See how many subtle movements and sensations you notice while practicing. Listen to the sound of your breath as you move through the rhythmical asanas. Feel your breath fuel your movements. In the stationary asanas, move your breath into the areas where you feel the greatest resistance to assist in releasing tension.*

TAKE FIVE (5 MINUTES)
- Complete Breath
- Spinal Flex II with Rotation
- Breath of Joy

SHORT PRACTICE (10 MINUTES)
- Complete Breath
- Spinal Flex II with Rotation
- Triangle
- Breath of Joy
- Arm Raise with Breath

MEDIUM PRACTICE (15-20 MINUTES)
- Complete Breath
- Spinal Flex II with Rotation
- Cobbler
- Half Dog
- Cow's Face
- Triangle
- Dancer
- Breath of Joy
- Arm Raise with Breath

"Changing Hats" – medium practice.

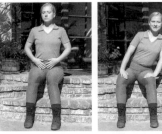
Complete Breath   Spinal Flex II

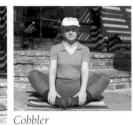
Cobbler

Half Dog

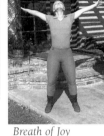
Cow's Face

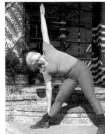
Triangle

Dancer

Breath of Joy

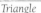
Arm Raise with Breath

This is a good opportunity to add:
• Meditation
• Visualization
• A mental rehearsal of your ride

SECTION 2. Yoga at the Stable

These routines were specifically chosen and adapted for practice at the stable in riding attire. When needed, use a mounting block, stable chair, fence, or the like to help in your warm-up. There are three separate warm-ups, each with a slightly different focus, but all balanced to stand on their own. Practice one favorite or alternate between them.

FLEXIBILITY

This practice focuses on increasing the flexibility of your muscles, ligaments, and joints. It includes a balanced selection of asanas to practice slowly, while you savor each stretch. Let time slow down throughout this routine as you pay particular attention to your breath. Deep and rhythmic breathing will enhance your ability to release tightness and relax more deeply into each asana, helping you stay aware of your edges. Spending increased time in each asana will help bring a deeper stretch to your muscles and tendons, creating greater flexibility over time.

REFLECTIONS: *Really* **relish** *each movement as you enjoy stretching through each asana in this practice. Imagine a cat stretching after a long nap in the sun. See if you can create that* *feeling of deliciousness and delight in each movement you make. Let your body express itself fully in each pose. Listen to the feedback you receive as you breathe and move. Take time to become reacquainted with your body and how it moves. Feel compassion and gratitude for all that your body does for you each day.*

TAKE FIVE (5 MINUTES)
- Spinal Flex II with Rotation
- Chest Expansion
- Two-Point Pose
- Straddle Fold and Rotation

SHORT PRACTICE (10 MINUTES)
- Spinal Flex II with Rotation
- Chest Expansion
- Two-Point Pose
- Dancer
- Triangle
- Straddle Fold and Rotation

MEDIUM PRACTICE (15-20 MINUTES)
- Spinal Flex II with Rotation
- Seated Camel
- Seated Twist
- Chest Expansion
- Two-Point Pose
- Dancer
- Triangle
- Straddle Fold and Rotation
- Symmetry

*"Flexibility" –
medium practice.*

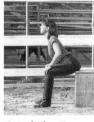

*Spinal Flex II
with Rotation*

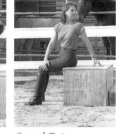

Seated Camel

Seated Twist

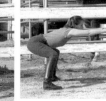

Chest Expansion

Two-Point Pose

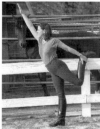

Dancer

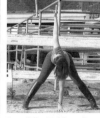

Triangle

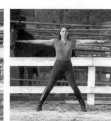

*Straddle Fold and
Rotation*

Symmetry

This is a good opportunity to add:
• A mental rehearsal of your ride

FOCUS

This dynamic practice sharpens mental focus and concentration using balance and breath and challenges particular muscles to engage while simultaneously maintaining relaxation in body and mind. This routine contributes to a strong sense of being grounded and connected to your Power Center; the perfect practice to explore your "sun/moon" polarities, such as maintaining a clear focus during dynamic activity while also feeling relaxed and fluid. As you combine these seemingly polar sensations, imagine experiencing them in balance on the horse.

REFLECTIONS: *Summon your personal power and intensity for this practice. The Warrior asanas were named for a mythical Indian warrior, Virabhadra, who was both strong and benevolent. While practicing, imagine you are a peaceful warrior, neither advancing nor retreating, but solidly holding your centered stance with intensity and compassion. Breathe with power and depth into your center, energizing your entire body with your breath as you fine-tune your balance. Focus ahead of you with intent while remaining receptive to the full space around you.*

TAKE FIVE (5 MINUTES)
• Arm Raise with Breath
• Triangle
• Dancer
• Centering Breath in Mountain

SHORT PRACTICE (10 MINUTES)
• Arm Raise with Breath
• Swayback
• Triangle
• Warrior I
• Dancer
• Centering Breath in Mountain

MEDIUM PRACTICE (15-20 MINUTES)
• Arm Raise with Breath
• Swayback
• Straddle Fold and Rotation
• Triangle
• Warrior I
• Dancer
• Half Eagle
• Cow's Face
• Centering Breath in Mountain

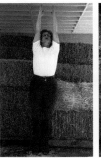 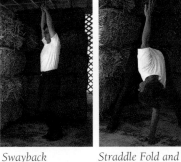 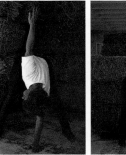 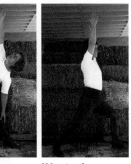

"Focus" – medium practice.

Arm Raise with Breath   Swayback   Straddle Fold and   Triangle   Warrior I

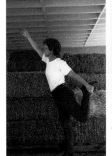 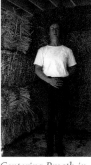

Half Eagle   Cow's Face

Dancer

Centering Breath in Mountain

This is a good opportunity to add:
• A mental rehearsal of your ride

FREEDOM

This practice encourages expansion and free movement. The asanas incorporate breathing synchronized with movement to build your awareness of rhythm. For riders who sometimes feel inhibited in their body or who experience energy blocks, difficulty relaxing on the horse, or just general tightness, this practice can set you free!

REFLECTIONS: *Put your heart into each movement and experience the natural flow of your body as you move in different ways. Push your usual edges of letting go. Activate the lines of energy in your practice and fully extend them in all directions. Expand, relax, and flow as you experience what it feels like to deeply release. Fill yourself with joy and freedom!*

TAKE FIVE (5 MINUTES)
• Spinal Flex II with Rotation
• Swinging Twist
• Breath of Joy
• Symmetry

SHORT PRACTICE (10 MINUTES)
• Spinal Flex II with Rotation
• Arm Raise with Breath

- Swinging Twist
- Chest Expansion
- Breath of Joy
- Symmetry

MEDIUM PRACTICE (15-20 MINUTES)

- Spinal Flex II with Rotation
- Shoulder Circles
- Arm Raise with Breath
- Swinging Twist
- Two-Point Pose
- Rhythmic Side Stretch
- Warrior II
- Breath of Joy
- Symmetry

This is a good opportunity to add:
- A mental rehearsal of your ride

"Freedom" – medium practice.

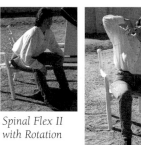

Spinal Flex II with Rotation

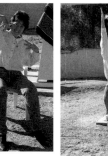

Shoulder Circles

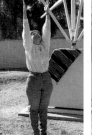

Arm Raise with Breath

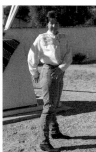

Swinging Twist

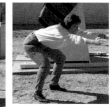

Two-Point Pose

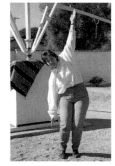

Rhythmic Side Stretch

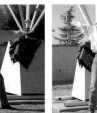

Warrior II

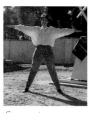

Breath of Joy

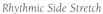

Symmetry

SECTION 3. Yoga at a Show or Competition

Preparing to ride in a horse show or competition adds to the routine business of warming up the rider's body the challenge of higher stress levels. The yoga techniques in this section can assist riders of different disciplines achieve the ability to relax, center, and focus—essential elements for a productive and fun show. If time allows, do one of the preceding yoga warm-ups *before* you arrive at the show grounds to make the following practices even more effective.

REFLECTIONS: *As you practice, let your breath help you "be in the moment." If your mind wanders, gently bring it back to the present by focusing on the sound and rhythm of your breathing. This is an excellent opportunity to use an affirmation or mantra, filling your mind with positive and constructive thoughts before showing.*

ENGLISH/JUMPING

In this English warm-up, begin with Alternate Nostril Breath, one of the most effective pranayama for quickly enhancing mental focus and bringing an overall equilibrium to your body and mind. The asanas efficiently tune your body by stretching your leg muscles and promoting fluid arms and shoulders and responsive and supple hips. Focus on balance and grounding to reinforce the feeling of connection you will need during your show ring performance, particularly over fences.

TAKE FIVE (5 MINUTES)
- Alternate Nostril Breath
- Chest Expansion or Two-Point Pose
- Grounding Exercise in Mountain

SHORT PRACTICE (10 MINUTES)
- Alternate Nostril Breath
- Half Dog Variation
- Warrior I
- Two-Point Pose
- Chest Expansion
- Grounding Exercise in Mountain

This is a good opportunity to add:
- A mental rehearsal of your ride
- Positive affirmations

English/jumping warm-up – short practice.

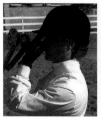

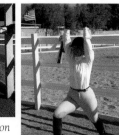

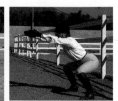

Alternate Nostril Breath

Half Dog Variation

Two-Point Pose

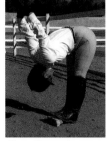

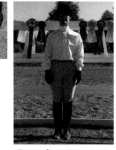

Warrior I

Chest Expansion (detail)

Chest Expansion

Grounding Exercise in Mountain

WESTERN

In this Western warm-up, we begin with Alternate Nostril Breath, excellent for dissipating stress or anxiety and bringing your mind into focus. Your range of movement may be inhibited somewhat by show clothes, so the routine does not require any extreme movements. The asanas bring fluidity to your arms and shoulders, supple your upper body so that it can move freely and independently throughout your competition, and stretch your hamstrings to encourage more freedom through your legs. By practicing the Centering Breath in Mountain, you can reinforce the sensation of being totally balanced and centered before you hop in the saddle. Try another Centering Breath before starting your competition.

TAKE FIVE (5 MINUTES)
- Alternate Nostril Breath
- Shoulder Circles
- Half Dog Variation
- Centering Breath in Mountain

SHORT PRACTICE (10 MINUTES)
- Alternate Nostril Breath
- Spinal Flex II with Rotation
- Seated Side Stretch
- Shoulder Circles
- Half Dog Variation
- Centering Breath in Mountain

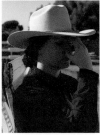

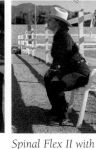

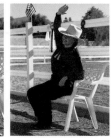

Alternate Nostril   Spinal Flex II with   Seated Side Stretch
Breath   Rotation

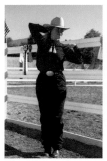

Shoulder Circles   Half Dog Variation   Centering Breath in
                                                  Mountain

Western warm-up – short practice.

This is a good opportunity to add:
• A mental rehearsal of your ride
• Positive affirmations

DRESSAGE

This dressage warm-up enhances your ability to quietly focus and stretch before your test. The practice starts with Alternate Nostril Breath, one of the most effective pranayama for quickly and effectively developing concentration and relaxing body and mind. The asanas promote long, independent, relaxed legs and open hips. They also help supple and stretch your back and shoulders, enabling you to follow the horse's movement without inhibiting it. Centering Breath in Mountain reinforces the sensation of being totally balanced and aligned before mounting. Once you have warmed up your horse, take another Centering Breath (with an assistant holding the reins) to regain this dynamic stillness before entering at "A."

TAKE FIVE (5 MINUTES)
• Alternate Nostril Breath
• Spinal Flex II with Rotation
• Warrior I Variation
• Centering Breath in Mountain

SHORT PRACTICE (10 MINUTES)
• Alternate Nostril Breath

- Spinal Flex II with Rotation
- Seated Twist
- Half Dog Variation
- Warrior I Variation
- Centering Breath in Mountain

This is a good opportunity to add:
- A mental rehearsal of your ride
- Positive affirmations

Dressage warm-up – short practice.

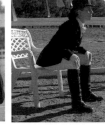

Alternate Nostril Breath

Spinal Flex II with Rotation

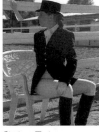

Sitting Twist

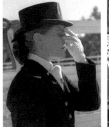

Half Dog Variation

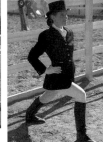

Warrior I Variation

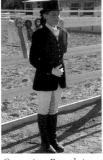

Centering Breath in Mountain

SECTION 4. Yoga After Riding

Few equestrians question the importance of cooling down their horse after a ride, but most riders neglect this essential practice when it comes to their own body. It is certainly easy to forget. We rightfully get occupied with caring for the horse first; by the time he is cooled off and put away, we have all but forgotten about the state of our own body. Until, perhaps the next day, when we feel some pangs of soreness or stiffness! There is no substitute for cooling down.

The following cool-down routines are easy and practical and assist in winding down from your riding activity, both physically and mentally.

About Cooling Down

Many riding activities are, to some degree, aerobic; your heart rate rises and blood concentrates in the muscles and extremities to fuel the physical demands of your riding. However, just as with the horse, going abruptly from a demanding ride to relative inactivity, especially in extreme weather conditions, can place undue stress on the body's systems, causing soreness. Taking the time to cool down gradually normalizes your heart rate and blood circulation, flushing the lactic acid generated during riding from the blood. If excess lactic acid remains in your muscles, it contributes to the soreness you may feel a day or two afterward.

If a cool-down is not currently part of your routine, you may need to exercise some creativity to find ways to include it. You will find that it is worth the effort. Begin your cool-down at the end of your ride by stretching your horse's back at the walk or trot. Ask the horse to lower his head and neck while maintaining relaxed forward movement to gradually wind down. This is an effective way to cool down together after a good work-out.

You also have other options. For example, utilize a groom or hot walker for five or ten minutes, and do one of the practices below as your horse is walked out. If you will be cooling out the horse yourself, enjoy walking together until you've both normalized. Then, as soon as you have a few minutes, do a short practice to keep your muscles supple and stretched.

If you end your ride abruptly (i.e., dismounting immediately as a reward), it is all the more important that you don't neglect your own cool-down. Make sure the horse is looked after, and then spend a good ten minutes on yourself. Once you start looking for ways to weave in some cool-down time for yourself, it is likely that you will find it. Get creative! You'll appreciate the rewards.

REFLECTIONS ON COOLING DOWN: *This is a time for winding down gradually. As you practice, begin to slow down your movements and the rhythm of your breath, providing your body time to relax. Breathe deeply and softly into all the asanas, enjoying the deep stretches. Hold them for as long as it feels good to you. This is also a good time to replay your ride in your mind. Appreciate yourself and the horse for the positive aspects of your time together. If there is anything you would do differently, take this time to visualize the changes you would make, seeing or feeling your ideal ride.*

COOL-DOWN 1

This cool-down enables you to control the pace at which you gradually slow your breath and movement, making it an ideal practice to follow a vigorous ride or immediately after dismounting. Take as much time as you need to wind down; once you have reduced your heart rate, enjoy the deep, relaxing stretches to finish.

VARIATIONS
- If your legs have had a particularly demanding workout in the saddle, try adding Warrior I or substituting Pyramid for Chest Expansion.

"In every state of training it is most important to ride for ten minutes at walk...after each session...by riding in walk at the end of the session you ensure that he [the horse] is breathing normally and taken back to his box [stall] in a physically and mentally relaxed condition."[90] PETRA AND WOLFGANG HÖLZEL AND MARTIN PLEWA, *Dressage Tips and Training Solutions*

• If you feel particularly overtaxed or excessively hot after your ride, avoid doing Chest Expansion, or any partial inversion, until you have normalized. Warrior I or Half Dog Variation are both effective substitutes.

TAKE FIVE (5 MINUTES)
• Rhythmic Side Stretch
• Spinal Flex II with Rotation
• Seated Twist
• Child's Pose

SHORT PRACTICE (10 MINUTES)
• Rhythmic Side Stretch
• Chest Expansion
• Spinal Flex II with Rotation
• Seated Twist
• Bent Willow
• Child's Pose

This is a good opportunity to add:
• Meditation
• A mental replay of your ride

Cool Down 1 – short practice.

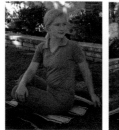

Rhymthic Side Stretch

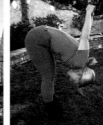

Chest Expansion

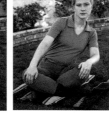

Spinal Flex II with Rotation

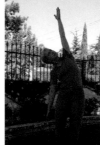

Seated Twist

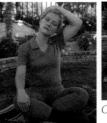

Bent Willow

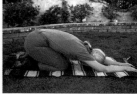

Child's Pose

COOL-DOWN 2

This practice keeps your body loose, giving good stretches to the muscles you have used in your ride to keep them long and supple. It increases awareness of the cadence of your breath, allowing you to gradually slow it down as your body's rhythms return to normal. This cool-down provides a deeper relaxation, enabling you to assimilate the prana you have generated. This will leave you feeling rested and rejuvenated!

VARIATION

- If you feel particularly overtaxed or excessively hot after your ride, avoid doing Straddle Fold (or any partial inversion, see p. 31) until you have normalized. Warrior I or Triangle are both effective substitutes.

TAKE FIVE (5 MINUTES)

- Swinging Twist
- Straddle Forward Fold and Rotation
- Horseshoe Stretch

SHORT PRACTICE (10 MINUTES)

- Swinging Twist
- Arm Raise with Breath
- Straddle Forward Fold and Rotation
- Horseshoe Stretch
- Centering Breath
- Corpse Pose

This is a good opportunity to add:
- Meditation
- A mental reply of your ride

Cool Down 2 – short practice.

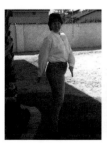
Swinging Twist

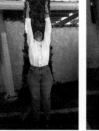
Arm Raise with Breath

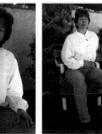
Straddle Forward Fold and Rotation

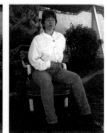
Horseshoe Stretch

Centering Breath

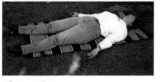
Corpse Pose

Yoga in the Saddle

"The chief motivator of our attitudes should be a love for the horses. When this theme encompasses all our intentions it fosters the humility and learning attitude which aid the rider to persevere through the difficulties encountered on the road to discovering the horse."[91] ERIK F. HERBERMANN, *The Dressage Formula*

YOGA IN THE SADDLE combines the principles of yoga with the moving and breathing energies of the horse. It is suitable for equestrians of any riding discipline. Used consistently, this program supports learning and complements any other riding instruction or training you receive on your journey toward Union. Before you perform the asanas and pranayama on the horse, please read through the "Guidelines for Mounted Practice" below and start with the preparatory exercises to engage your breath and imagination.

Time with Your Horse

Yoga in the Saddle enhances the valuable skills already gained from your unmounted yoga practice. Know that this is a precious time to include your equine partner in your practice. When you spend time with your horse practicing Yoga in the Saddle, pay close attention to your body and all that you feel. Notice how the horse's body feels underneath you. This focused and revitalizing time provides a wonderful opportunity for deepening your connection with the horse, as well as with your inner self. Delight in experiencing and exploring the many sensations, thoughts, and feelings that emerge as you practice Yoga in the Saddle.

The asanas that follow have been adapted for horseback and provide a very special and unique benefit for the rider: the opportunity to blend the practice of yoga with riding a horse! As you practice, you may develop enhanced levels of relaxation and connectedness with the horse, finding that you can more easily maintain these qualities throughout your ride.

GUIDELINES FOR MOUNTED PRACTICE

- The majority of yoga guidelines apply to practice both in and out of the saddle. The safety of both horse and rider is essential to good horsemanship and should be observed at all times.

- Although it's not a prerequisite, it is beneficial to practice the unmounted versions of the asanas and pranayama before attempting them in the saddle.

- Proper riding attire and protective headgear are recommended for all mounted activities. Avoid wearing loose-fitting hats or sunglasses that may fall off while practicing.

- Use the tack you normally ride with; these exercises can easily be performed in all types of English, Western, or dressage saddles. Ensure that your saddle is comfortable and fits both you and the horse correctly.

- Yoga in the Saddle is ideally performed on a quiet, cooperative horse, at the halt or walk, with the help of an assistant or trainer to hold or lead the horse as necessary. If possible, practice on a longe line under the supervision of a riding instructor. With someone else monitoring the direction and speed of the horse you are riding, you will feel more relaxed and secure, able to perform the mounted yoga mindfully.

- Begin your practice by sitting balanced and centered in the saddle. Establish your grounding connection with the horse and the earth, simultaneously lengthening upward from your Power Center. Your feet can either be in or out of the stirrups.

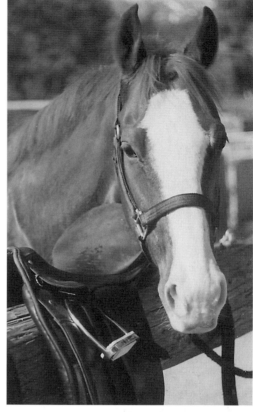

Yoga in the saddle is a great way to nurture the partnership you share with the horse.

- Be mindful of how the horse may react to the movements of your torso, arms, hands, and legs while you are mounted. Move consciously to avoid spooking the horse as you move into each position.

- You may practice either with your eyes closed to assist in focusing your attention inward, or with your eyes open, focusing softly to maintain awareness of your surroundings.

- Yoga in the Saddle can also be practiced bareback, allowing for an even closer connection with the horse. Maintaining a secure balance, without relying on grip, is essential. Be especially mindful of not startling the horse as you place your hands on his body for support. To avoid mishaps, we strongly recommend that bareback riders adhere to all safety guidelines and not practice yoga on the horse without supervision or assistance.

The next exercise will help you relax throughout your entire body while increasing awareness of your Power Center. Use your enhanced awareness to gently align your pelvis in an upright, vertical position. With practice, you will feel centered in all aspects. Centering Breath is a great way to prepare for riding and can be helpful as a brief "time out" during times of frustration in a lesson, before going into the show ring, or any time you need to regain a sense of calm. Have someone read the following exercise and visualizations aloud as you begin at the halt with an assistant holding the horse's head.

MOUNTED AWARENESS EXERCISE: Centering Breath

RECOMMENDED GAIT: HALT

1. Sit comfortably on the horse, your weight distributed evenly on both seat bones. Place your dominant hand on the front of your body one to two inches below your navel. Place your other palm against your lower back to encircle your Power Center between both hands. Close your eyes and take several deep breaths.

2. Think of your hands as possessing a magnetic pull to draw your breath down into your Power Center. Breathe slowly and deeply, inhaling through your nose and exhaling through your mouth. As you inhale, allow your abdomen to expand under your dominant hand. As you exhale, use that hand to assist the abdominals in pushing out all the air. Feel this entire area become energized as it expands and contracts with each Centering Breath.

3. On an exhalation, purposefully engage your abdominals inward and upward to assist in aligning your pelvis. Lower your back hand to your sacrum and guide it into a more vertical position, directing your seat bones toward the front of the saddle. Breathe deeply as your lower body sinks into the horse. Do not tense the muscles of your of your lower body to push yourself deeper into the saddle—let gravity take you.

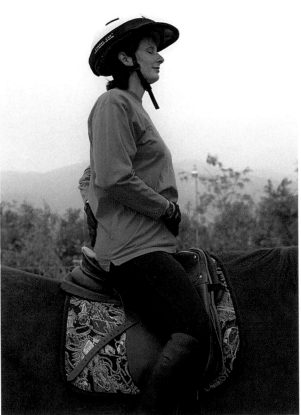

Centering Breath.

4. Let your legs hang, lightly draped around the horse's sides, your ankles and feet relaxed. Dropping your stirrups will increase the stretch in your legs, although you may keep them if you prefer, lightly resting the balls of your feet on the stirrups.

5. Keep breathing fully into your Power Center with an even, regular tempo as you reposition your hands lightly on your thighs, pommel, or saddle horn. Allow your arms and shoulders to relax and hang down. Imagine that you are wearing a heavy cape across your shoulders; feel its weight across your upper back.

6. Continue to breathe deeply, while softening and widening your lower back. From your Power Center, become aware of your spine stretching both up and down. Inhale and feel your spine extend upward from your Power Center. Hold that upward stretch through your torso as you exhale, then feel your spine extend downward. Pause to experience this sensation and take several deep breaths before continuing on.

7. Allow your breath to fill your entire body with each inhalation. Listen to the sound of your breath as it carries tension out of your body. Feel your hip joints release as your seat deepens. Relax your legs so that they drop even lower as you soften your knee and ankle joints. Your body now feels relaxed, aligned, and secure in the saddle.

Now that your body is well positioned on the horse, this grounding visualization will help anchor you, deepening the connection with the horse and the earth.

MOUNTED VISUALIZATION: **Earth**

RECOMMENDED GAIT: HALT

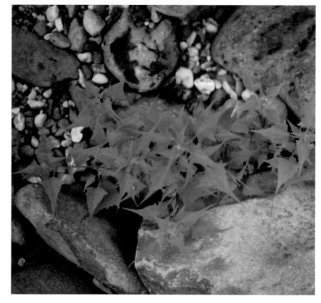

With your eyes closed, breathe deeply into your Power Center. See a column of energy that runs down through the base of your spine, your seat bones, the saddle, and into your horse's body. Let your lower body stretch toward the earth as you exhale. Feel your center of gravity in alignment with your horse's center of gravity, the energy from your spine blending with the energy in his spine. Feel his spinal cord surge underneath your seat with power and sensitivity. Notice...your spine and his are mere centimeters apart.

Connect with the Earth. (Photo: Veronica Wirth)

See and feel your column of energy flow through your horse into the ground below, then deep into the earth, anchoring you. Pause to enjoy the sensation of increased stability in the saddle as you feel more united with your horse. Take several deep breaths before continuing on.

Gravity has grounded your body with the horse and down into the earth. The following visualization will help you reach for the sky to align with the greater energy above you.

MOUNTED VISUALIZATION: **Sky**

RECOMMENDED GAIT: HALT

Stretch toward the sky. (Photo: Veronica Wirth)

To begin, reaffirm your grounding connection and awareness of your Power Center. With a deep inhalation, lighten your upper body and allow your spine to elongate upward toward the sky. Breathe space between each vertebra, aligning each one atop the other. As you exhale, hold this lightness in your upper body while simultaneously stretching your lower spine down into the horse. Continue lengthening your upper body with each inhalation and grounding downward with each exhalation.

As your body lengthens upward, imagine a column of energy traveling up through your spine from your Power Center. Let this energy pass between your shoulder blades and up through the back of your neck. Allow your head to feel weightless, balanced effortlessly over your spine. Increase the space between the last vertebra (the atlas), and your head.

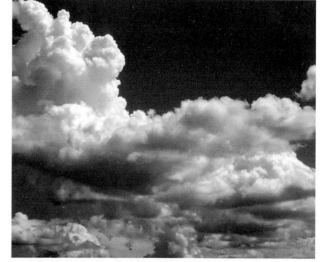

Feel your head floating freely upward and imagine the top of your head opening up to the sky. Send the column of energy up through the top of your head and connect it to the greater energy above you. Imagine a shining gold sphere above your head, or see your energy column connect to a star or the sun. The prana is now moving freely both up and down your spine. Pause once again to enjoy the feeling of connection within yourself, to your horse, to the earth and sky. Take several deep breaths before continuing on.

ALTERNATE NOSTRIL BREATH

RECOMMENDED GAIT: HALT

RIDER BENEFITS: Excellent for relieving anxiety and creating a sense of calm. Promotes emotional stability essential for riding. Ideal for a general rider warm-up or before going into the show ring. This fundamental pranayama deepens the rider's breath, and assists in balancing, centering, and focusing the mind.

TIP: To fully understand the sequence, read through all of the steps before beginning. As you count, keep a slow tempo throughout.

1. Begin sitting quietly at the halt. With a deep inhalation, extend upward from your Power Center. As you exhale, ground down through your seat, your legs draped loosely around the horse's sides.

2. Using your right hand, rest your thumb lightly on the right side of your nose, your forefinger and middle finger lightly between your eyebrows, your ring and pinkie finger lightly on the left side of your nose (see photo detail, p. 39).

Alternate Nostril Breath.

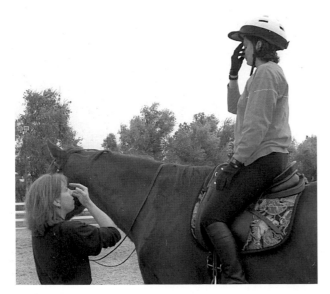

3. Close your right nostril with your right thumb, inhale deeply through your left nostril to a count of 4. Keeping your right nostril closed, close the left nostril with your ring and pinkie fingers, and hold your breath for a count of 4. Release your thumb and exhale completely through your right nostril.

4. Without pausing, your left nostril still closed, inhale deeply through your right nostril to a count of 4. Close your right nostril and hold for a count of 4. Then release your left nostril and exhale fully for a count of 4. This completes one full cycle of Alternate Nostril Breath. The steps are clarified as follows:

Inhale, left nostril 4 counts
Hold inhalation 4 counts (both nostrils closed)
Exhale, right nostril 4 counts
Inhale, right nostril 4 counts

Hold inhalation 4 counts (both nostrils closed)

Exhale, left nostril 4 counts

5. Complete 4 full cycles. As this breath becomes easier, you can increase the number of cycles.

TIPS FOR TRAINERS OR ASSISTANTS: Assist the rider by *slowly* counting each step, for example "Inhale right, 2, 3, 4, hold 2, 3, 4, etc." Remind the student to relax her legs, release her hips, and keep her shoulders relaxed down. This pranayama can be performed with eyes open or closed; if the rider is uncomfortable or starts to lose balance with their eyes closed, suggest that they gaze softly at the horse's neck.

TRIANGLE

RECOMMENDED GAIT(S): HALT OR WALK

RIDER BENEFITS: Assists in suppling and stretching the rider's sides uniformly in both directions. Also encourages the rider to keep her hips straight, weight distributed evenly on both seat bones. Triangle in the saddle will help the rider maintain a secure, balanced lower body, encouraging independent movement of the upper body.

Triangle.

1. With a deep inhalation, place your right hand on your right knee; sweep your left arm out to the side and up overhead. Breathe deeply and rhythmically. Keep your left elbow and wrist straight and ensure that your weight is evenly distributed on both seat bones.

2. Stretch through your entire left side while reaching your left arm toward the opposite side. Keep your arm energized all the way to your fingertips. Relax your legs, grounding down through your seat bones as you enjoy the stretch all along your left side. Watch that you don't fall forward through your left shoulder and arm or collapse through your right waist. Imagine your upper body is between two panes of glass (one in front and one behind you) to assist in keeping your arms, shoulders, and spine aligned.

3. Hold for 4 deep breaths, then release back to the center, lowering your left arm as you exhale. Repeat to the left.

4. To finish, come back to center and take a few centering breaths before moving on.

TIPS FOR TRAINERS OR ASSISTANTS: At the walk, remind the rider to breathe in rhythm with the movement of the horse. While the rider's arm is extended overhead, remind her to breathe intercostally, lifting upward through her rib cage so that she does not collapse at the waist. Ensure that the rider stretches from her Power Center both upward and downward through the spine.

CAMEL

RECOMMENDED GAIT: HALT

RIDER BENEFITS: Camel provides an excellent stretch for the front of the body, opening the chest and releasing shoulder tension. Improves flexibility and strengthens the rider's back. Creates a significant opening through the ribs and chest, allowing for a more complete use of lung capacity.

1. Breathe deeply and center. On an exhalation, place both hands on the cantle as you relax your entire lower body and draw your shoulders down away from your ears.

2. As you inhale, lift and open your chest to the sky, gradually arching your middle and upper back. Drawing your shoulders back and down, gently allow your head to tip back, following the curve of your spine. (If you have any pain or discomfort in your neck, keep your head and eyes forward.) Stay balanced on both seat bones and lift up from your Power Center. With your pelvis anchoring you in the saddle, allow for a slight pelvic tilt as your lower back flexes to follow the entire spinal arc. Let your arms help support the weight of your torso.

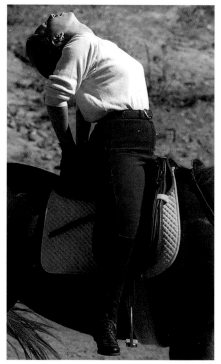

Camel.

3. Exhale and reaffirm that you are grounded down into the horse and the earth as your upper body relaxes further into this backward bend. With each breath, feel your intercostal muscles expand and your chest open and reach toward the sky; stretch upward from your lower back.

4. Stay here for several deep and relaxed breaths. When you are ready to release the pose, keep your hands on the cantle to support you while you slowly roll your upper body upward, one vertebra at a time, until you are fully upright. Breathe and center to finish.

COUNTER-POSES: Chest Expansion, Half Eagle, or bend forward and hug the horse around his neck!

TIPS FOR TRAINERS OR ASSISTANTS: As this pose provides a profound stretch to the rider's torso with the head drawn back, ensure that it is performed at the halt under supervision. Emphasize lifting from the Power Center, which is more important than how much the rider can arch her back. It is imperative to avoid compressing the lumbar vertebrae, which commonly results from too much arch in the lower back. Ensure that the rider keeps her hands on the cantle to gently support her upper body should the horse shift his weight or move suddenly. If bareback, the rider can carefully place her hands behind her, on either side of the horse's spine. Remind the rider to breathe fully!

CHEST EXPANSION

RECOMMENDED GAIT: HALT

RIDER BENEFITS: Chest Expansion draws the shoulder blades together, creating expansion in the rider's chest, helping to establish balance and alignment in the upper body. The forward bend accentuates the stretch and increases the release of the rider's shoulders, while encouraging the back and neck muscles to soften.

1. Clasp your hands together behind your back. Take a deep intercostal breath, opening your chest and bringing your shoulder blades closer together. With your shoulders rolled back and down, feel your chest widen and open as you stretch upward through your torso.

2. On an exhalation, bend forward from your Power Center, rounding your spine and letting your arms and clasped hands reach up toward the sky. Remain balanced and centered, keeping a light contact with your seat bones in the saddle.

3. With each inhalation, lift more with your hands and arms, expanding your chest. Roll your shoulders back. With each exhalation, allow gravity to take the weight of your upper body down toward the horse's neck.

4. Hold this asana for several breaths. Slowly and gently come back into an upright, full-seat position in the saddle.

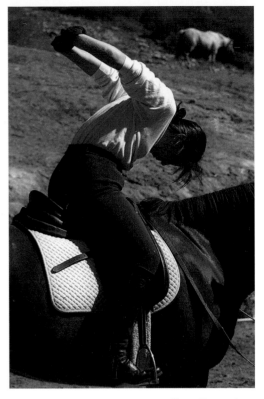

Chest Expansion.

TIPS FOR TRAINERS OR ASSISTANTS: Remind the rider to stay centered and balanced evenly on both seat bones, both legs dropping evenly down around the horse's barrel. Do not allow the rider to press her body into the pommel, saddle horn, or the horse's neck. Remind the rider to release her neck and allow her head to hang down while bending forward. When coming upright, advise the rider to roll back up slowly, one vertebra at a time.

TWIST

RECOMMENDED GAIT(S): HALT OR WALK

RIDER BENEFITS: Excellent for developing symmetrical suppleness in the back while it teaches the rider to stretch and lengthen upward, rotate the torso laterally, and open the chest. Increases flexibility and suppleness in the lower and middle back, enhancing the rider's ability to receive the horse. Further balances and aligns the spine while encouraging centered awareness on the horse.

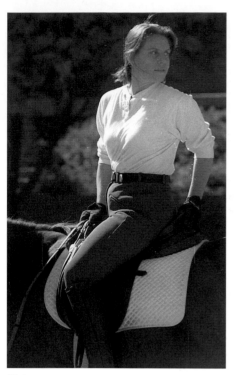

Twist.

1. Inhale deeply and stretch up from your Power Center; sit evenly in the saddle with your arms relaxed by your sides.

2. As you exhale, place your left hand on the pommel or horn of your saddle and your right hand on the cantle.

3. With a deep inhalation, stretch up through your spine and turn to look over your right shoulder toward your horse's hindquarters. Feel your spine softly rotate all the way through your body, from your evenly weighted seat bones to your head.

4. As you exhale, allow your body to relax and open into the twist. Find the degree of rotation that feels good to you. Let your arms lightly support you but do not force the twist. Remain here for several full breaths, continuing to stretch upward from your Power Center with each inhalation, softly opening into the twist with each exhalation.

5. To finish, let go with your hands and gently unwind your body to face forward once again. Pause in the starting position for a moment and take a few breaths, then repeat this asana to the left, reversing your hands as you look over your left shoulder.

TIPS FOR TRAINERS OR ASSISTANTS: If Twist is performed at the walk, remind the rider to keep her hips moving in rhythm with the horse's motion; if the pelvis becomes immobilized, the horse may halt. To avoid compression of the lower spine, ensure that the rider stretches upward as she inhales, deepening the twist and extending down through her lower body with each exhalation, never forcing. Bareback riders should exercise care when touching the horse's back and avoid placing any direct pressure on the horse's spine. As the rider looks over her shoulder, suggest the use of a focal point. To increase the stretch, encourage the rider to look slightly beyond her focal point. (Using a visual point of reference will also assist the rider in becoming aware of her progress.)

TWIST WITH ARMS EXTENDED

RECOMMENDED GAIT(S): HALT OR WALK

RIDER BENEFITS: Supples the rider's back, encouraging uniform rotation in both directions. Increases the upward stretch while adding a horizontal stretch through extended arms. The rider is challenged to remain centered while directing energy outward through her arms and experiencing the vertical flow of energy through her spine. Teaches the torso to move independently of the lower body and to initiate movement from the Power Center.

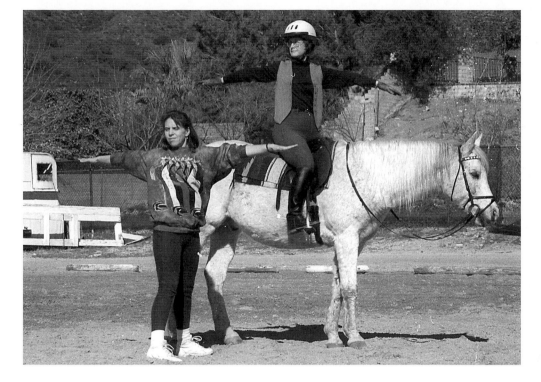

Twist with Arms Extended.

1. Inhale deeply, extending your arms straight out to each side. Stretch up through your spine and outward through your arms, hands, and fingers. Keep your arms extended straight out from your shoulders. Feel a strong flow of energy running horizontally through your arms and out your extended fingertips. Maintain the vertical line of energy that extends from your Power Center.

2. As you exhale, twist to your right, looking over your right shoulder past your fingertips, toward the back of your horse. Feel the rotation of your spine extending from your seat bones all the way to your head. Allow your seat and legs to sink deeply. Let the exhalation assist you in deepening into the twist. Be aware of the extension of your arms out to the sides. Keep your weight evenly distributed between both seat bones. Adjust your seat if necessary.

3. As you inhale, rotate forward to the center with your arms still out to each side. Repeat to the left. Twist at least 4 times to each side. When performed at the halt, your movements should be fluid and correspond to the natural rhythm of your breath. At a walk, your movements and breathing should match the tempo and rhythm of your horse's gait.

4. To finish, return to starting position, take a deep breath, and let your arms softly float down as you exhale. Breathe here and center before moving on.

TIPS FOR TRAINERS OR ASSISTANTS: At the walk, remind the rider to breathe in rhythm with the movement of the horse, matching both twisting and breathing to the walk rhythm. (If the rider's pelvis becomes immobilized, the horse may halt.) Encourage the rider to keep her lower back supple and relaxed. Ensure that the rider experiences both vertical and horizontal stretches in her body. Prompt the rider to keep her arms energized by reaching out through the fingertips, activating the horizontal line of energy.

HALF EAGLE

RECOMMENDED GAIT: HALT

RIDER BENEFITS: Loosens the joints of the elbows and shoulders and brings a deep stretch to the upper torso. Also provides isometric strengthening of forearms, wrists, and hands. Ideal for riders who carry tension in their upper or middle back; helps break up muscle knots and tightness.

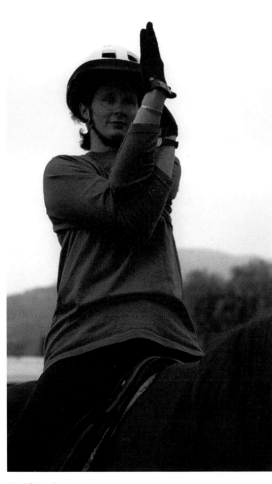

Half Eagle.

1. Face forward and take a few deep, intercostal breaths as you grow tall and light through your upper body. Choose a focal point in front of you. Release your hips and allow your seat to relax and widen, enabling you to sit deeper in the saddle.

2. Center your right arm in front of you, bending your elbow. Point your forearm straight up with a flat palm facing left.

3. Wrap your left arm under your right elbow, bringing it straight up on the right side, palm facing right.

4. Bring the fingers of your left hand to rest on the palm of your right hand. If this is a difficult reach for you, try linking a finger with your thumb. Adjust the degree of stretch by either lowering or raising your elbows.

5. Gaze straight ahead, past your arms, and breathe deeply into your Power Center. Direct your breath into the space between your shoulder blades, consciously releasing tension there with each exhalation. Hold for at least 4 deep breaths. Gradually work your way up to 8 breaths or more.

6. Release your arms slowly and consciously, stretching them in any way that feels good. Reverse your arm position and repeat.

TIPS FOR TRAINERS OR ASSISTANTS: To help the rider release the space between her shoulder blades, place your hand on this area and encourage her to "breathe into your hand." Advise the rider to adjust the degree of stretch by raising or lowering her elbows. If the rider cannot touch her hands together, have her bring them as close as possible, fingers pointed straight up.

COW'S FACE

RECOMMENDED GAIT: HALT

RIDER BENEFITS: Helps break up tension and increases range of motion in the rider's upper back, shoulders, and elbows. This stretch enhances the independent use of the rider's arms and encourages the spine to align, the chest to open, and shoulders to draw back, counteracting the common rider habit of rounding the back and collapsing forward. Increases breathing capacity by opening the chest.

TIP: Use readily available props such as a lead rope, crop, towel, or riding glove, etc.

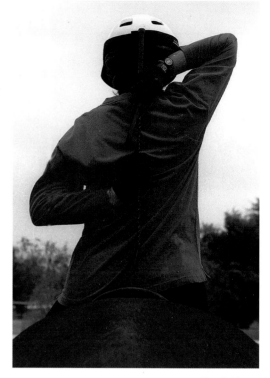

Cow's Face.

1. Lengthen through your upper body; open your chest and bring your shoulders back and down. From your Power Center, feel your lower body melting down into your horse.

2. Reach behind your back with your left arm, placing your left hand as far up on your spine as you comfortably can.

3. With a deep inhalation, stretch your right arm straight up over your head. Bend your elbow and let your hand reach down toward the center of your back, palm down. Can your hands touch each other? If so, hook your fingers or grasp hands, depending on your level of flexibility. If not, use a prop to bridge the gap.

4. Gently move your hands closer together to increase the stretch. Listen closely to your body and respect your edges. Remember to breathe!

5. Gaze straight ahead and take several intercostal breaths to open and lift your chest. Stretch your elbows straight up and down; relax your shoulders as much as you can to help them release and open. With each breath, lighten, release, and expand! Hold for at least 4 deep breaths. Gradually work your way up to 8 breaths or more.

6. Come out of this pose slowly and consciously. Shake out your arms and repeat on the opposite side; stretch and shake out again. Breathe and center.

TIPS FOR TRAINERS OR ASSISTANTS: Have a prop available before the rider begins this pose. Make sure that the rider looks forward, keeping her upper body elongated and aligned, chest open. Suggest the elbows stretch in both directions, activating this vertical line of energy to keep the elbows in alignment.

✦

A New Path

YOGA FOR EQUESTRIANS advocates an approach to riding that encourages understanding, patience, and compassion for horse and rider. An instructor who teaches in this manner can inspire you to successfully pursue your riding dreams. Treating your own body according to this approach expands the possibilities for success as you cultivate your skills in a safe, pleasurable, and progressive manner. Whether you ride for pleasure, sport, or art, Yoga for Equestrians offers a new learning path and guides you to integrate your body and mind with those of the horse. This fresh, inspiring program can help transform unfavorable habits into favorable ones along the path to the fulfillment of your riding goals and dreams.

Integrating yoga practice with your riding will improve your ability to understand the horse's silent body language while you cultivate a parallel ability to better understand the language of your own, often *unknown*, inner landscape. Along the way to becoming a better rider, you are faced with many external variables. But within you lie variables "hidden from view." These are perhaps the trickiest to identify, address, and modify. Becoming aware of your inner self is one key to developing heightened self-mastery that can lead to Union.

As you sit astride your horse, listen with your body. Notice his desire to find balance with you. By nature, horses are generally willing to please once you have earned their trust and exhibit a gratifying tendency toward seeking Union with you. Honor the horse by striving to become the best rider you can be. The horse will reflect the positive qualities, insights, and knowledge that you acquire and serve you faithfully.

The time may come when you notice that your riding habits have changed. The boundaries between you and your horse begin to blur. You may discover that "suddenly" you are able to breathe deeply and smoothly in a situation that previously caused you to hold your breath. Perhaps you will become conscious of deep relaxation while you ride in sync with the horse. When these realizations occur, let your spirits soar in celebration of this powerful sense of Union.

Your new skills may occasionally slip during the periods of difficulty, frustration, or stress that trigger your body and mind to instinctively revert to old, ingrained habits and responses. Do not be discouraged, but embrace it as a natural part of your learning process. Persevere and continue to trust yourself and your developing skills. Know that with practice, you will consistently establish relaxation, flow, and connection with the horse.

Yoga for Equestrians is a circular process; each accomplishment, each step you take along your journey, both requires your participation as a whole being and affects you in your totality. As you become balanced, inside and out, your entire being becomes more unified and connected. In realizing the benefits of yoga practice, you will grow to understand and welcome this circular process of discovery that guides you toward wholeness in all that you do.

The most important thing to remember while practicing Yoga for Equestrians is to HAVE FUN! Like riding, yoga is a gift you give to yourself. Allow the qualities of your yoga practice to heighten the experiences of discovery, awareness, depth, and delight that enrich your time spent with horses. We think you will find that yoga and riding will nurture one another, nourishing your body, mind, and spirit in the process.

~ Namaste ~

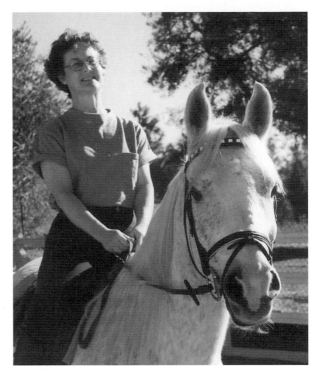

Acknowledgments

From Us Both

To Martha Cook and Caroline Robbins at Trafalgar Square Publishing, our deepest thanks to you for extending this opportunity to us as first-time authors. We are so grateful for your patience, knowledge, and guidance throughout the process of birthing this book—you helped make our vision a reality! Thank you to our copyeditor, Sue Ducharme, for your keen eye and ability to draw out the essence of our ideas. To Elizabeth Carnes at Half Halt Press, we thank you for steering us in the right direction and greatly appreciate your personal referral.

To all our students, thank you! In particular, we would like to give special thanks to those who have helped us beyond the call of duty: Virginia Hildreth, for your invaluable feedback, generous participation, wholehearted support of the program, and extraordinary enthusiasm; Dena Phillips, for your graphic talents and support, and working your magic on that Mac! Apryl Knobbe, thank you for your dedication and participation; Marguerite Norton, we're grateful for your enthusiasm and assistance.

To all our friends, students, and riders who photographed so beautifully, both on and off the horse: Heidi Baumgarten, Jaynetta Christian, Erica Chuang, Amanda Deaton, Gerardo Espitia, Dennis Fallon, John Grote, Virginia Hildreth, Mimi Yan Henderson, Apryl Knobbe, Lindsey and Steven Martin, Marguerite Norton, Dena Phillips, Edie Reaves, Bettina Roth, Anna Ruth Souza, and Diane Yurkas.

For the insightful student interviews we thank Apryl Knobbe, Anna Ruth Souza, Virginia Hildreth, Amanda Deaton, and Sarah Rose.

To our technical advisors: Douglas B. Grisier, D.O., Patrick St. John, D.C., and Edie Reaves, Certified Massage Therapist. Thank you for your qualified review of our anatomical research and for your helpful recommendations. We appreciate the time you spent, your knowledge of the human body, and your enthusiasm for the book.

Thanks to Karen Boras and Martha Hernandez for so generously letting us use your space and your computers and enabling us to create a dedicated writing sanctuary. And thanks to Helena Wirth for extending her space to us during the editing period of this manuscript. We are especially grateful to all of you for your hospitality and kindness. To Val Mehling, thank you for your technical assistance, computer know-how, and for lending us one when we really needed it. To Art Martinucci, for your professional counsel and guidance. In light of your many obligations, we thank you for the time you graciously volunteered to assist us.

To everyone who has assisted us in each step along the way, we are most grateful.

From Veronica

I offer my sincere gratitude to my yoga students who continue to teach me through their courage to discover their own wisdom.

Mom, how can I ever thank you? There is no way I could have done this without your bottomless love and support. You constantly show me that love knows no boundaries. Your wisdom, courage, fortitude, and inner peace inspire me. For this, and so much more, I am eternally grateful. Thank you with all my heart!

My deepest gratitude is extended to my teachers and mentors. Brian Bennett, for always being there with your wise and gentle insight, for knowing all along that I could do this, and for teaching by example. I am so blessed to count you as both a friend and a teacher. Becky Loving, fellow Taurean! Thank you for your generous guidance, joyful wisdom, and for inspiring me to always see the bigger picture.

Ganga White and Tracy Rich of the White Lotus Foundation, thank you for sharing your wisdom so generously, and for the beautiful space you have created to share it in!

To all my dear friends and kindred spirits—I am grateful for your much valued support, wisdom, empathy, patience, and understanding. You kept me sane and helped me see the light through uncharted territory.

From Linda

Gerardo, mi amor...gracias por toda tu ayuda y apoyo. Nunca hubiera podido escribir este libro sin tu asistencia. Eres el amor de mi vida y te amo mucho. Se que ahora, una puerta se está abriendo hacia una nueva vida para nosotros.

To my family and friends on the East coast and across the country, my deep appreciation for the support and interest you've shown throughout the years toward all of my artistic and equestrian endeavors. To my family of friends on the West coast, many thanks for helping me create a sense of community, for your companionship, and the good times we've shared, as these have all contributed to my ability to remain strong and committed to my dreams. A special thanks to Deb for your support, your words of wisdom, and for always being just a phone call away when I needed you!

Thanks to Paul Gilbert who passed away before the completion of this book. He was a man who loved horses and once told me that I had restored his faith in humankind. Paul, I am grateful for having had the opportunity to work with you and your horses at the ranch, and for developing my program there...it was never the same without you. Peace to you.

To Simone Lagomarsino and the Olive View Equestrian Center, thanks for the beautiful grounds that were used as backdrops for many of our photo shoots; and to you we offer our infinite gratitude for generously assisting Harmony With Horses amidst the chaos of our relocation. Your immaculate facility and concern for the horses is both admirable and refreshing.

Thanks to my riding students throughout the years and especially to those who have been an integral part of the Harmony With Horses program. I am so proud of you all and I can't tell you how exciting and fulfilling it has been for me to share your equestrian journeys.

Finally, thanks to all my teachers, including my equine partners, especially Radar (my CEO—Chief Equine Officer), Buddy (our cover horse), Pele, Peggy, Cherokee, Vicar; and all the private and lesson horses that have willingly assisted me in teaching others and have been patiently teaching me all along.

Glossary

Aerobic—describes physical activity that increases heart rate over a period of time, improves respiration, increases consumption of oxygen, and conditions the body.

Affirmation—A positive statement made in the present tense that asserts something to be true. Used as a mantra to foster a meditative state of mind so that the positive statement may more easily be assimilated by the subconscious mind to effect desired changes in riding and yoga practice.

Altered State—An uncommon state of mind or an experience of consciousness that differs from your ordinary state. Generally, a state of wakeful relaxation in which the brain's electrical wave patterns decrease from the beta rhythm associated with normal consciousness (13-30 cycles per second) to the slower alpha rhythm (8 to 13 cycles per second). See Rhythmic Stillness and Union.

Articulates—To unite by a joint. This term is used to accurately describe the relationship between jointed skeletal structures. For example, the sacrum articulates with the pelvis at the sacroiliac joint.

Asana—A Sanskrit word meaning "posture." Ancient poses practiced in Hatha yoga that balance, tone, and integrate body, mind, and spirit, creating overall good health and well-being.

Atlas—The first cervical vertebra (C1), which supports the weight of the skull, named after a Titan in Greek mythology who was forced by the gods to bear the weight of the world on his shoulders.

Axis—The second cervical vertebra (C2). So named because it articulates with the atlas and forms the pivot upon which the head and atlas move. Together, the first two vertebrae permit the rotation and nodding movements of the head.

Balanced Seat—Also known as the vertical seat, the classical seat, the full seat, the three-point position, the riding asana. Position is sustained through a rider's balance, as opposed to grip; based on the vertical alignment of the rider's entire spine over a sturdy base of support. An upright pelvis supports and stabilizes this position. For general riding, the rider's legs are in contact with the horse and positioned so that the heels and hips are aligned with large, open angles at the hips and knees, the heel lower than the toe. Most commonly used by dressage and Western riders, the principles of the balanced seat are easily adapted to other disciplines.

Beginner's Mind—A receptive state of mind that perceives any situation as being fresh, or brand new. Also referred to as an "open mind" or "empty cup." Involves setting judgment and predispositions aside to ensure the mind is uncluttered, ready to receive information objectively.

Body Memory—The autonomic function of the body that results in memory of physical and emotional information that is stored on a cellular level. Relevant to the process of integrating physical positions or movements while learning a new skill. In the event of trauma or injury to a specific area, the memory of pain which persists beyond the initial incident, often triggering the body's protective responses.

Body-Mind—Refers to a person's body and mind as one cohesive unit, each aspect affecting the other.

Cadence—Rhythmic, sequential quality of movement or sound made up of a regular, fluid measure of beats. Is especially relevant to breathing and work at the trot.

Carpal Tunnel Syndrome—In the wrist, the carpal tunnel houses the median nerve and the flexor tendons. Strain or inflammation caused by repetitive motion or overbending of the wrist can cause irritation to tendons and nerves, resulting in pain, numbness, and tingling. A widespread syndrome due to the common use of computers and other repetitive machines in the workplace; can also result from incorrect use of the wrists while riding.

Center—Also called the physical center. A point in the body located about two inches below the navel and just in front of the lumbar spine. See Power Center. *v.* To center is the act of focusing inward to both quiet the mind and balance the body. To "come back to center" is to return to your starting position in a pose or exercise—**centering.**

Center of Gravity—Also known as center of mass. The central point within a body where its weight is concentrated. If supported at this spot, the body remains in perfect balance in any position.

Centered—A quality reflecting relaxed focus and composure in mind and body.

Conscious Rider—An open-minded, responsible equestrian committed to growth, who approaches riding with awareness, perception, and purpose.

Consciousness—Your state of mind. To elevate consciousness is to increase awareness of, and be open to, absorbing internal or external information. To be mentally unconscious is to be unaware, unable, or unwilling to learn or receive information.

Counter-pose—A complementary asana to balance the opposing group of muscles to those actively used in an asana involving intense bend, stretch, etc. Part of a well-rounded practice intended to balance opposing muscles groups and avoid injury or overworking muscles.

Edge(s)—That fine line between going too far in your work and not going far enough. Becoming sensitive to your edges should not involve pain. A fluid, change-able boundary that may be affected by physical, mental, emotional, or spiritual factors.

Energy—see **Prana**

Energy Center—A component of your Power Center that stores, regulates, and conducts the flow of prana inwardly and outwardly through your body. The energy center is located deep in your abdominal area (Sphere of Influence) and corre-sponds to your physical center. Also referred to as the *hara*.

Energy-Block—An area of the body where energy or prana is restricted. May be due to chronic tension or injury; inhibits movement through that area of the body.

Feminine Energy—Energy that produces personal attributes characterized as feminine in nature, such as receptivity, intuition, nurturing, sensitivity. These feminine aspects are complemented by their masculine counterparts. Both aspects are present in each individual to varying degrees.

Fight or Flight Mechanism—A primitive, involuntary release of adrenaline in response to an actual or perceived threat. When faced with a situation which the nervous system perceives as life-threat-ening, results in either preparation for doing battle or flight.

Flow Experience—An optimal experience

or altered state wherein time seems to stand still and activity flows effortlessly. Involves being intensely focused in the moment while engaging in a proficient level of activity experienced with no obstructions.

Frame—*n.* The position, shape, or silhouette of either horse or rider created by the skeletal support structure and the musculature that surrounds it. The quality of the frame refers to the posture of the body and how the body is carried. *v.* To frame the horse refers to the rider's ability to influence a desirable posture, or carriage, in the horse's body.

Grounding—*v.* To establish a powerful sensation of stability and connection to the surface beneath your body through visualization and directing the breath. For example, when standing, "grounding through your feet" means to direct energy from your Power Center down your legs and feet, through the floor and into the earth, imagining you are growing roots. *n.* A grounding cord is a mental tool you imagine or feel, to anchor you to what is below.

Hara—see **Energy Center**

Hatha Yoga—The path of yoga that creates balance in body, mind, and spirit through the practice of physical postures and stretches called asanas and breathing techniques called pranayama.

Holistic—Concerned with the whole. Perceiving and treating the Self as a complete system rather than a collection of parts. A holistic approach to health or activity requires understanding the interrelatedness of all aspects of each living being (e.g., horse and rider) with the ultimate goal of achieving overall balance.

Isometric—A muscular contraction occurring against resistance but without the shortening of the muscle or movement of the bone(s) that results in a substantial increase in muscle tone.

Isotonic—A muscular contraction occurring without resistance but with significant shortening of the muscle and movement of the bone(s), without much increase in muscle tone.

Kinesthetic—Describes the ability of the rider's body to perceive the condition, alignment, and placement of the body in relationship to its surroundings, to movement, and to the horse. Kinesthetic information becomes body memory, allowing the rider to ride and respond to the horse with an increasingly instinctive feel. See Body Memory.

Lines of Energy—Pathways that channel energy from the Power Center through "lines" created by the spine, arms, and legs; activated with awareness and fueled by the breath; produced in both stationary postures and movement.

Mantra—Fundamentally, the repetition of an idea, thought, or concept usually expressed through sound; a word or phrase used to focus the mind and induce a meditative state. An organic mantra is a vital, rhythmical repetitive movement such as breathing, walking, or riding used to achieve rhythmical stillness.

Masculine Energy—Energy that produces attributes deemed masculine in nature, such as leadership, activity, assertiveness, strength. These masculine aspects are complemented by their feminine counterparts; both are present in each individual in varying degrees.

Metronome—A device that produces regularly repeated clicks to mark a steady beat. Used in learning to keep an even tempo in music and sometimes in riding.

Meditation—The act of stilling, quieting, and clearing the mind to foster enhanced states of relaxation, awareness, and receptivity in both mind and body.

Mirroring—The horse's ability to reflect qualities of the rider's interaction, which appear as either desirable or undesirable behaviors in the horse.

Polarities—Opposite, complementary, or contrasting qualities such as light/dark, push/yield, active/passive, feminine/masculine, etc.

Power Center—The regulator of physical movement and energy throughout the body. Location of the corresponding physical and energetic centers of the body.

Prana—The life-force or universal energy that is present in every living thing.

Pranayama—Yogic breathing exercises that generate and regulate the flow of prana through the body. By increasing lung capacity, building strength and control of the breath, pranayama fortify the inherent link between body, mind, and spirit.

Release—The act of freely "letting go" without excessive effort or stress. With respect to muscles, it means to relax and stop "holding on," allowing the muscle to become as soft and free as possible. With regard to emotions, it refers to allowing a feeling to freely move through you.

Rhythm—A regular pattern or arrangement of recurring movement or sound. For example, the horse's walk has a four-beat rhythm, corresponding to the pattern of each leg sequentially striking the ground, one at a time.

Rhythmic Stillness—An integrated, harmonious state of mental focus and physical proficiency achieved through a rhythmical activity, either on or off the horse. In riding, it describes a rider's ability to be fully present, in a state of quiet concentration, while engaged in the dynamic, physical activity of riding. Rhythmic Stillness is a type of altered state experienced on the horse.

Sanskrit—The language of the ancient, sacred texts of India, called the Vedas.

Self—A term used to represent the unified elements that comprise the identity of an individual: physical, emotional, mental, and spiritual. When used as a prefix, "self" indicates a quality or item belonging to, or relating to, the individual such as self-awareness; self-knowledge.

Self-Carriage The ability to maintain proper balance and alignment, with minimal strength and effort, independent of artificial means or incorrect position. This term applies to both rider and horse, describing the efficient usage of the physical body which, in self-carriage, expresses poise and grace through movement.

Soul—see **Spirit**

Sphere of Influence—The central section of a rider's body physically comprised of supporting structures—such as the pelvis, seat bones, lumbar spine, and sacrum—and the musculature of the abdominals and lower back. Together, these features can be thought of as a "sphere" that influences a rider's ability to center, balance, and maintain upright alignment both on and off the horse. The Power Center is housed within the Sphere of Influence.

Spirit—The soul or energetic aspect of Self, also referred to as higher-self or higher-consciousness. Refers to the aspect of Self that has the ability to assimilate or comprehend knowledge and wisdom that surpasses the mundane.

Stillness—A meditative state of interior quiet and peace, where mental chatter is erased and the body is relaxed.

Supine—Lying down; flat on one's back; reclining; horizontal.

Tempo—The rate of speed of a rhythmical movement, sound, or activity. In the horse, lack of tempo is exhibited when "lagging behind" or "rushing" his gaits.

Union—The dynamic, harmonious integration of body, mind, and horse attained through skillful riding; an altered state, flow experience, or rhythmic stillness experienced on the horse. Often, a spiritual unity evolving from a rider's high level of awareness and self-mastery, coupled with the horse's increased willingness and focus. As the boundaries between horse and rider become blurred, both partners exhibit a mutual ability to merge, becoming One, achieving Union.

Visualization—The natural act of using the imagination to create mental visual images.

Weight Shifting—Subtle, inconspicuous aids involving controlled displacement of weight occurring in the rider's lower body, usually on the seat bones, without disrupting upper body integrity. Used in balancing, straightening, and flexing the horse; executing turns, lateral movements, etc.

✦

Resources

Harmony With Horses Enterprises

THE BALANCED RIDING PROGRAM OF SOUTHERN CALIFORNIA
This unique, holistic program is the birthplace of *Yoga for Equestrians* and is dedicated to the development of conscious, balanced, harmonious riders – recreational, competitive, amateur, or professional. Directed by Linda Benedik, a classical instructor of the balanced seat, riding lessons are integrated with hatha yoga to aid in "sculpting" a rider's position and to encourage awareness and self-mastery. To more clearly interpret the ideals of horsemanship, Linda presents a compassionate, progressive method and inspires equestrians to approach their journey patiently and mindfully to ride with greater ease, more feel, and a rhythmical synchronicity with the horse. Her insightful instruction also blends elements of music, art, dance, breathwork, and bodywork and offers a fresh approach to achieving traditional goals.

Private Clinics and Riding Holidays feature unmounted RiderHarmony™ Workshops, longe-line lessons, "Yoga in the Saddle," instruction in balanced seat riding, traditional equitation, and classical dressage on schoolmasters from Intro Level to FEI. Workshops introduce "rider groundwork" and may include pranayama, asanas, walking meditations, guided visualizations, riding theory, and horsemanship. The mutual relaxation of rider and horse is emphasized and programs are tailored to the individual.

Weekend Riding Clinics begin with a Friday evening unmounted RiderHarmony™ Workshop that combines the principles of classical riding with a gentle, beginner-level yoga practice geared toward equestrians. Two full days of riding lessons complete the program. Participants will learn how to maintain a relaxed, coordinated rhythm on the horse through various gaits, transitions, lateral movements, and arena patterns. Linda will work with riders on the longe line to facilitate a secure seat and balanced position. Her integrated clinics have been enjoyed by riders of many disciplines including dressage, eventing, English, Western, reining, trail, endurance, and vaulting.

Harmony With Horses Dressage offers an integrated, classical approach to the art and discipline of dressage. *Dressage*, from the French word *dresser* means "to train," and, when correctly applied, can improve the performance of any horse. By patiently cultivating a deep secure seat, vertical position, coordination of the aids, sensitivity, suppleness, a focused calm, and rhythmical breathing with movement on the horse, riders can progressively achieve a state Linda calls "RiderHarmony" This essential mind-body balance is key to achieving positive training results with the horse and for demonstrating a rider's comprehension of the purpose and requirements of each level.

Our programs continue to evolve and grow. For more information, please contact:

Harmony With Horses Enterprises
Linda Benedik, Founder & Director
Post Office Box 1107, Ventura, CA 93002-1107, USA
Toll Free: 877-419-0399 (Pacific Time)
24-Hour Voice Mail: 805-243-9943
e-mail: riderharmony@earthlink.net
web site: www.harmonywithhorses.com

Veronica Wirth - Certified Yoga Instructor

You are invited to join me in ongoing instruction on Yoga for Equestrians, and intuitive Hatha yoga in the Southern California area. My teaching synthesizes yoga, meditation, breathwork, channeling, healing, and energy work in a very gentle and supportive atmosphere. Private and semi-private sessions are offered, tailoring our work together to address your unique goals and dreams. Classes and workshops are available upon request.

I am available to travel nationally and internationally to give individual instruction, group classes or workshops, and healing.

To find out more details on the above, as well as new developments, please contact me at the information below. I would be delighted to hear from you!

Veronica Wirth
2497 Park Row East
Montreal, Québec H4B 2H8
Canada
Tel: 514-483-8996
e-mail: vwomanyoga@yahoo.co.uk

YOGA RESOURCES (USA)

Bheka Yoga Supplies
474 Applegate Way
Ashland, OR 97520
Tel: 800-366-4541
www.bheka.com

Hugger Mugger Yoga Products
3937 So. 500 W.
Salt Lake City, UT 84123
Tel: 800-473-4888
www.huggermugger.com

YogaMats
P.O. Box 885044
San Francisco, CA 94188
Tel: 800-720-YOGA
www.yogamats.com

Yoga Zone
3 Park Plaza
Old Brookville, NY 11545
Tel: 800-264-9642
www.yogazone.com

YOGA RESOURCES (UK)

Ruth White's Yoga Centre
Tel: 020 8644 0309
www.ruthwhiteyoga.com

British Wheel of Yoga
Tel: 01529 306 851
www.bwy.org.uk

The Yoga Shop
Tel: 0870 066 4202
www.theyogashop.co.uk

Eye Yoga
Tel: 0870 014 0310
www.eyeyoga.co.uk

PUBLICATIONS

Yoga Journal
Tel: 800-600-YOGA
www.yogajournal.com
An excellent yoga resource

Yoga International
Tel: 800-253-6243
email: yimag@yimag.com
A yoga magazine published in the US
and distributed internationally

Yoga and Health Magazine
Tel: 01273 565 111
www.yogaandhealthmag.co.uk
A monthly journal published in the UK

APPENDIX 3

References

PART I

1. MÜSELER, WILHELM, *Riding Logic* (New York: Simon and Schuster, Inc., 1983, p. 9).

Chapter 1

2. XENOPHON, *The Art of Horsemanship*, translated by Morris H. Morgan, Ph.D. (London: J.A. Allen & Company, Ltd., 1962)

Chapter 2

3. MOHAN, A.G., *Yoga for Body, Breath, and Mind* (Portland, OR: Rudra Press, 1993, p.12).
4. SIVANANDA YOGA VENDANTA CENTER, *Yoga Mind and Body* (New York: DK Publishing, Inc., 1996, p.6).
5. PIERCE, MARGARET D. AND MARTIN G., *Yoga for Your Life* (Portland, Oregon: Rudra Press, 1996, p.10).
6. MOHAN, A.G., *Yoga for Body, Breath, and Mind* (Portland, OR: Rudra Press, 1993, p.13).
7. MOHAN, A.G., *Yoga for Body, Breath, and Mind* (Portland, OR: Rudra Press, 1993, p.13).
8. SCHIFFMANN, ERICH, *Yoga: The Spirit and Practice of Moving Into Stillness* (New York: Pocket Books, a division of Simon & Schuster, 1996, p.3).
9. SCHAEFFER, RACHEL, *Yoga for Your Spiritual Muscles* (Wheaton, Illinois: Theosophical Publishing House, 1998, p.2).
10. COUCH, JEAN, *The Runner's Yoga Book* (Berkley, CA: Rodmell Press, 1990, p.7).
11. OHLIG, ADELHEID, *Luna Yoga* (Woodstock, New York: Ash Tree Publishing, 1994, p.32).
12. Hassler, Jill Keiser, Beyond the Mirrors (Quarryville, PA: Goals Unlimited Press, 1988, p.108).
13. ACKERMAN, SHERRY L., *Dressage in the Fourth Dimension* (Cleveland Heights, OH: Xenophon Press, 1997, p.52).

Chapter 3

14. KRAMER, JOEL, "Yoga as Self-Transformation," Yoga Journal, (May/June 1980)
15. WALTON, TODD, Open Body, Creating Your Own Yoga (New York: Avon Books, 1998, p.65).
16. We must credit GANGA WHITE, of the White Lotus Foundation, for this delightful analogy! From *Yoga Teacher Training*, 1998.
17. SCHAEFFER, RACHEL, *Yoga for Your Spiritual Muscles* (Wheaton, Illinois: Theosophical Publishing House, 1998, p.6).

PART II

18. ACKERMAN, SHERRY L., *Dressage in the Fourth Dimension* (Cleveland Heights, OH: Xenophon Press, 1997, p.29).

Chapter 4

19. FARHI, DONNA, *The Breathing Book* (New York: Henry Holt & Company Inc., 1996, p.53).
20. FARHI, DONNA, *The Breathing Book* (New York: Henry Holt & Company Inc., 1996, p.5).
21. *Ibid.*, p.5.

22. CARRICO, MARA, *Yoga Journal's Yoga Basics* (New York: Owl Books, 1997, p.43).
23. CATHERINE PONDER, *Open Your Mind to Receive* (Marina Del Rey, California: DeVorss & Co., 1983, p.26).
24. BENNETT, BIJA, *Breathing Into Life* (New York: HarperCollins Publishers, 1993, p.xiii).

Chapter 5
25. MARCINIAK, BARBARA, *Earth* (Santa Fe, New Mexico: Bear & Company, Inc., 1995, p.84).
26. SAVOIE, JANE, *That Winning Feeling* (North Pomfret, Vermont: Trafalgar Square; Publishing, and in UK: J.A. Allen & Co. Ltd, 1992, p.7).
27. SILVA, JOSÉ, *The Silva Mind Control Method* (New York: Simon & Schuster, Inc., 1977, p.61).
28. HASSLER, JILL KEISER, *Beyond the Mirrors* (Quarryville, PA: Goals Unlimited Press, 1988, p.79).
29. VISHNUDEVANANDA, SWAMI, *The Complete Illustrated Book of Yoga* (New York: Bell Publishing, 1960, p.221).
30. SIVANANDA YOGA VENDANTA CENTER, *Yoga Mind and Body* (New York: DK Publishing, Inc. 1996, p.156).
31. LESHAN, LAWRENCE, *How to Meditate* (Boston, Massachusetts: Little Brown & Company, 1974, p.29).
32. SCHIFFMANN, ERICH, *Yoga: The Spirit and Practice of Moving Into Stillness* (New York: Pocket Books, a division of Simon & Schuster, 1996, p.306).
33. BENSON, M.D., HERBERT, *The Relaxation Response* (New York: William Morrow and Company, Inc., 1975, p.111).
34. GAWAIN, SHAKTI, *Creative Visualization* (New York: Bantam Books, 1978, p.2-3).
35. *Ibid.*
36. KRAMER, JOEL, "Yoga as Self-Transformation," *Yoga Journal*, (May/June 1980).
37. ROMAN, SANAYA, *Spiritual Growth* (Tiburon, CA: HJ Kramer, Inc., 1989, p.35).
38. CARRICO, MARA, *Yoga Journal's Yoga Basics* (New York: Owl Books, 1997, p.167).
39. CSIKSZENTMIHALYI, MIHALY, *Flow* (New York: HarperCollins Publishers, 1990, p.21).
40. SCHIFFMANN, ERICH, Yoga: *The Spirit and Practice of Moving Into Stillness* (New York: Pocket Books, a division of Simon & Schuster, 1996, p.46).
41. MCCORMICK PH.D., ADELE VON RÜST AND MARLENA DEBORAH, *Horse Sense and the Human Heart*, (Deerfield Beach Florida: Health Communications, Inc., 1997, p.xx).
42. STRICKLAND, CHARLENE, *Western Riding* (Pownal, Vermont: Storey Communications, Inc., 1995, p.66-68).
43. BLAZER, DON, *Natural Western Riding* (Boston, Massachusetts: Houghton Mifflin Company, 1979, p.42).
44. HASSLER, JILL KEISER, *Beyond the Mirrors* (Quarryville, PA: Goals Unlimited Press, 1988, p.122).
45. ACKERMAN, SHERRY L., *Dressage in the Fourth Dimension,* (Cleveland Heights, OH: Xenophon Press, 1997, p.19).
46. CSIKSZENTMIHALYI, MIHALY, *Flow* (New York: HarperCollins Publishers, 1990, p.41).
47. *Ibid.,* p.42.
48. HASSLER, JILL KEISER, *Beyond the Mirrors* (Quarryville, PA: Goals Unlimited Press, 1988, p.122).
49. DE KUNFFY, CHARLES, *Dressage Questions Answered* (New York: Arco Publishing, Inc., 1984, p.9).

PART III
50. ACKERMAN, SHERRY L., *Dressage in the Fourth Dimension* (Cleveland Heights, OH: Xenophon Press, 1997, p.37)

Chapter 6
51. HILL, CHERRY, *Becoming an Effective Rider* (Pownal, Vermont: Storey Communications, 1991, p.24).

52. SCARAVELLI, VANDA, *Awakening the Spine* (New York: HarperCollins Publishers, 1991, p.101).
53. SWIFT, SALLY, *Centered Riding* (North Pomfret, Vermont: Trafalgar Square Publishing, 1985, p.134).
54. HILL, CHERRY, *Becoming an Effective Rider* (Pownal, Vermont: Storey Communications, Inc., 1991, p.70).
55. SWIFT, SALLY, *Centered Riding* (North Pomfret, Vermont: Trafalgar Square Publishing, 1985, p.10).
56. SMITH, BOB, *Yoga for a New Age* (Engelwood Cliffs, New Jersey: Prentice-Hall, Inc., 1982, p.27).
57. WALTON, TODD, *Open Body* (New York: Avon Books, 1998, p.58).
58. MÜSELER, WILHELM, *Riding Logic* (New York: Simon & Schuster, Inc., 1983, p.46-47).
59. WANLESS, MARY, *Ride With Your Mind* (North Pomfret, Vermont: Trafalgar Square Publishing, 1991, p.151).
60. *Ibid.*, p.40.
61. SMITH, BOB, *Yoga for a New Age* (Engelwood Cliffs, New Jersey: Prentice-Hall, Inc., 1982, p.30).
62. HILL, CHERRY, *Becoming an Effective Rider* (Pownal, Vermont: Storey Communications, Inc., 1991, p.155,160).
63. SMITH, BOB, *Yoga for a New Age* (Engelwood Cliffs, New Jersey: Prentice-Hall, Inc., 1982, p.30).

Chapter 7

64. SCHIFFMANN, ERICH, *Yoga: The Spirit and Practice of Moving Into Stillness* (New York: Pocket Books, a division of Simon & Schuster, 1996, p.25).
65. *Ibid.*, p.48.
66. HOLMES, TOM, *The Total Rider* (Boonsboro, MD: Half Halt Press, Inc; and in the UK: Kenilworth Press, 1995, p.3)
67. *Ibid.*
68. MÜSELER, WILHELM, *Riding Logic* (New York: Simon & Schuster, Inc., 1983, p.17).
69. COUCH, JEAN, *The Runner's Yoga Book* (Berkeley, CA: Rodmell Press, 1990, p.79).
70. DE KUNFFY, CHARLES, *Dressage Questions Answered* (New York: Arco Publishing, Inc., 1984, p.184, 191).
71. LUBY, THIA, *Children's Book of Yoga* (Santa Fe, New Mexico: Clear Light Publishers, 1998, p.10).

Chapter 8

72. SCARAVELLI, VANDA, *Awakening the Spine* (New York: HarperCollins Publishers, 1991, p.28).
73. COUCH, JEAN, *The Runner's Yoga Book* (Berkeley, CA: Rodmell Press, 1990, p.113).
74. PODHAJSKY, ALOIS, *The Complete Training of Horse and Rider* (North Hollywood, California, Wilshire Book Company, 1967, p.213).
75. SMITH, BOB, *Yoga for a New Age* (Engelwood Cliffs, New Jersey: Prentice-Hall, Inc., 1982, p.30-31).
76. SCHAEFFER, RACHEL, *Yoga for Your Spiritual Muscles* (Wheaton, Illinois: Theosophical Publishing House, 1998, p.92).
77. TOTTLE, SALLY A., *BodySense* (North Pomfret, Vermont: Trafalgar Square Publishing; and in the UK: Kenilworth Press, 1998, p.32).
78. BALASKAS, JANET, *Preparing for Birth with Yoga* (Great Britain: Element Books, 1994, p.146).
79. SCARAVELLI, VANDA, *Awakening the Spine* (New York: HarperCollins Publishers, 1991, p.48).
80. DE KUNFFY, CHARLES, *Dressage Questions Answered* (New York: Arco Publishing, Inc., 1984, p.196).
81. SWIFT, SALLY, *Centered Riding* (North Pomfret, Vermont: Trafalgar Square Publishing,

1985, p.47).

82. GRAY F. R. S., HENRY, *Anatomy of the Human Body* (Philadelphia: Lea & Febiger, 1950, p.78).

83. *Ibid.*, p.79.

84. SMITH, BOB, *Yoga for a New Age* (Engelwood Cliffs, New Jersey: Prentice-Hall, Inc., 1982, p.34)

85. SCARAVELLI, VANDA, *Awakening the Spine* (New York: HarperCollins Publishers, 1991, p.8).

86. LASATER, PH.D., P.T., JUDITH, *Relax and Renew* (Berkeley, CA: Rodmell Press, 1995, p.89).

87. SMITH, BOB, *Yoga for a New Age* (Engelwood Cliffs, New Jersey: Prentice-Hall, Inc., 1982, p.34).

88. ACKERMAN, SHERRY, L., *Dressage in the Fourth Dimension* (Cleveland Heights, OH: Xenophon Press, 1997, p.26).

PART IV

89. MCCORMICK PH.D., ADELE VON RÜST AND MARLENA DEBORAH, *Horse Sense and the Human Heart*, (Deerfield Beach Florida: Health Communications, Inc., 1997, p.210).

Chapter 9

90. HÖLZEL, PETRA AND WOLFGANG, AND MARTIN PLEWA, *Dressage Tips and Training Solutions* (North Pomfret, Vermont: Trafalgar Square Publishing; and in the UK: Kenilworth Press, 1995, p.9).

Chapter 10

91. Herbermann, Erik F., The Dressage Formula (London: J.A. Allen & Company Limited, 1984, p.23).

Quick-Reference Guide
to Asanas, Pranayama, and Exercises

ALPHABETICAL LISTING
+ indicates mounted version

AWARENESS EXERCISES

Breathe Into Your Back, p.115-116
+ Breathing and Riding, p.44-45
+ Centering Breath, p.68; + p.162-163
Find Your Sacrum, p.77-78
Weight Shifting, Part I, p.82-83
Weight Shifting, Part II, p.83

MEDITATION

The Sound of Your Breath, p.52-53

VISUALIZATIONS

Clearing Energy Blocks, p.54
+ Earth p.163
Grounding, p.81
Intertwine Your Energy with the Horse, p.70
Lines of Energy, p.55-56
Mental Rehearsal of Your Ride, p.56-57
Power Center, p.67-68
+ Sky, p.163-164
Skyward Energy Flow, p.131-132

SUBJECT GUIDE

LEGS

Chest Expansion
Forward Fold, Standing
Forward Fold, Straddle
Pyramid
Side Stretch, Rhythmic
Swayback
Toe Touch
Triangle
Two-Point Pose
Warrior I
Warrior II

SPINE

Breathe Into Your Back
Cat Stretch
Dancer
Forward Fold, Standing
Forward Fold, Straddle and Rotation
Spinal Flex I and II with Rotation
Twist, Seated

HIPS

Bridge
Cobbler
Dancer
Forward Fold, Straddle
Happy Baby
Pyramid
Triangle
Twist, Seated
Warrior I
Warrior II

PELVIS

Cat Stretch
Cobbler
Earth
Grounding
Swayback

ABDOMINALS

Abdominal Lift
Boat
Bridge
Oblique Strengthener
Toe Touch

SEAT

Abdominal Lift
Bridge
Cobbler
Earth
Find Your Sacrum
Grounding
Happy Baby
Pyramid
Swayback
Toe Touch
Triangle
Warrior I
Warrior II

BALANCE

Dancer
Grounding
Mountain

BALANCE (CONT.)
Swayback
Triangle
Warrior I
Warrior II

ALIGNMENT
Clearing Energy Blocks
Earth
Forward Fold, Straddle and Rotation
Lines of Energy
Mountain
Side Stretch, Seated
Sky
Symmetry
Triangle
Warrior I
Warrior II

BREATHING
Abdominal Lift
Alternate Nostril Breath
Arm Raise with Breath
Breath of Joy
Breathe Into Your Back
Breathing and Riding
Complete Breath
Intercostal Breath
Spinal Flex I and II with Rotation
The Sound of Your Breath

BREATHING WITH RHYTHM AND MOVEMENT
Arm Raise with Breath
Breathing and Riding
Bridge
Cat Stretch
Side Stretch, Rhythmic
Spinal Flex I and II with Rotation

ARMS AND HANDS
Arm Raise with Breath
Breath of Joy
Cow's Face
Eagle, Half
Reverse Namaste
Twist, Swinging

SEAT BONE AWARENESS
Cobbler
Earth
Easy Pose
Grounding
Weight Shifting, Part I and II
Side Stretch, Seated
Spinal Flex I and II with Rotation

HEAD AND NECK
Bent Willow
Forward Fold, Standing
Hare
Horseshoe Stretch
Sky
Skyward Energy Flow
Twist, Swinging

SHOULDERS AND UPPER BACK
Arm Raise with Breath
Breath of Joy
Chest Expansion
Cow's Face
Dancer
Dog, Quarter and Half
Eagle, Half
Forward Fold, Standing
Hare
Reverse Namaste
Shoulder Circles

CENTERING
Arm Raise with Breath
Centering Breath
Complete Breath
Dancer
Earth
Grounding
Intertwine Your Energy with the Horse
Mental Rehearsal of Your Ride
Mountain
Power Center
Sky
Symmetry
The Sound of Your Breath

Index

Main entries appear in **bold** type